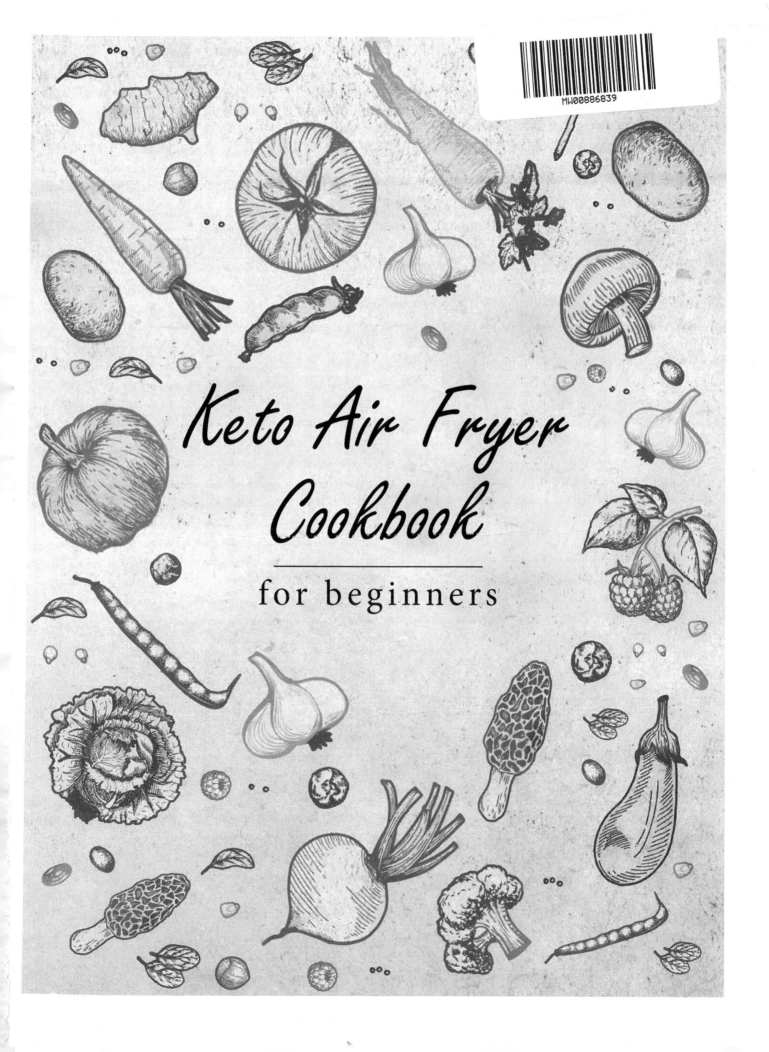

Keto Air Fryer Cookbook

for beginners

Contents

Introduction

According to a study in Obesity Reviews, approximately 42 percent of adults globally are trying to lose weight. The Boston Medical Center claims that in the United States alone, some 45 million people go on diets each year and collectively spend $33 billion per year on products to assist them. The point is that you're not alone. You are not the only person struggling to lose weight.

There are many reasons why weight loss is so hard, but one of the most common is that dieting is difficult to maintain. Without getting too scientific here, for some people, the brain has been hardwired to respond positively to unhealthy foods. You know that mushy feeling you get when you think about that big juicy cheeseburger? Well, that's your brain firing out the feel-good hormone dopamine. Once that feeling kicks in, it's difficult to shake and you're either making your way to the drive through or ordering a takeaway. To begin, eating salads just doesn't have the same effect, but what people don't know is that if they stuck it out, they would.

What I've just described used to be my problem. Most people don't believe me when I tell them that five years ago, I weighed 350 lbs! Yep, I sure did. I was overweight, a borderline diabetic with chronic back pain and a host of other health problems. But today, I weigh 160 lbs and I'm completely healthy. What happened? The ketogenic diet!

I spent years trying to lose weight, every year I made the same New Year's Resolution – that I would shed the pounds and start taking care of my body. I would go on one of the many fad diets that are conveniently pushed in our faces at the beginning of the year and give up within a week because I couldn't control my cravings. It wasn't until I got introduced to the keto diet that I felt hopeful. "Finally," I thought to myself, "a diet that actually allows me to eat." To be honest, I thought it was too good to be true until I started seeing the weight fall off.

The rapid weight loss, high energy, clear focus, and diminishing health problems not only motivated me to keep going but made me curious about the science behind the diet which led me to start reading about it. As a result, I've spent the past five years rigorously studying the ketogenic diet, and the more I learned, the more I believed in it.

Keto isn't a fad, it's a lifestyle. Thousands, perhaps millions of people globally are choosing to eat this way because it has so many benefits (all of which you can read about in the next chapter).

Whether you're already on the keto diet, or you're just getting started, you chose this book because you need some recipe inspiration, but I can promise you, you'll get a lot more than recipes. Here are some of the things you can learn:

- The food you can and cannot eat
- The benefits of the keto diet
- The benefits of using an air fryer to cook
- Mouth-watering vegetarian recipes
- Succulent sea food recipes
- Delicious desserts
- And much more

Are you ready to make a commitment and change your life for the better? Are you ready to shed some pounds, reclaim your physical power and become the person you were destined to be? If so, keep reading...

Chapter 1: Keto Diet and Air Fryer Explained

The ketogenic diet, also known as, 'keto,' is a low-carbohydrate, high-fat diet. Although it's gained popularity over recent years, the diet isn't new. Medical practitioners used it during the nineteenth century to treat diabetes, but it's famously known for treating epilepsy in children. Non-traditional doctors have also treated conditions such as Alzheimer's disease, polycystic ovary syndrome, and cancer with the ketogenic diet. Nevertheless, recently, the diet has gained a lot of attention because of its extreme weight-loss capabilities. Low-carb diets such as Atkins, Dukan, South Beach and Paleo have put low-carb diets on the map. But keto seems to be leading the pack. What is it that makes this diet so special?

What is the Keto Diet?

The idea is that if the body is starved of glucose from carbohydrates, which is the main energy source for the cells, it will start burning fat for energy instead. The evidence proves that this works because when there are not many carbohydrates available, the body goes to glucose reserves stored in the liver. But to achieve this, it has to break down muscle. It takes between 3 and 4 days for the body to use all the stored glucose which then causes a decrease in insulin levels and the body is forced to use fat as its energy source. When there's no glucose, the liver uses fat to make ketone bodies. As these ketones increase, the body goes into a state of ketosis and turns into a fat burning machine.

Dieters cannot consume more than 50 grams of carbohydrates per day. Keeping carbohydrate intake low is the most important aspect of the diet. There are no specific measurements for protein and fat intake, but most popular resources recommend around 75 grams of protein, and 165 grams of fat. You'll find several versions of the ketogenic diet out there, but they're all low carb. Additionally, there are slight variations on food lists, but the key is to stick to the diet until you've reached your desired weight loss goal.

Food You Can Eat and Food You Should Avoid

While it's true that you can still eat a lot of your favorite foods on the keto diet, it's still very restrictive. As you'll soon read, there are some healthy foods that are off limits or that you can only eat in small amounts. But first, let's start with the foods you can eat.

Meat and Eggs

Beef	Sardines	Eggs
Chicken	Albacore tuna	Pork
Turkey	Salmon	

Fruits and Vegetables

Broccoli	Avocado	Green beans
Bell peppers	Zucchini	Cauliflower
Berries	Spinach	

Dairy

Sour cream	Plain Greek yogurt	Cheese
Heavy cream	Butter	Cottage cheese

Miscellaneous

Unsweetened plant-based milks	Unsweetened coffee and tea	Cocoa powder
Nuts and seeds	Alternative flours	
Olive oil	Dark chocolate	

Nuts and Seeds: These are the best nuts and seeds to eat on the keto diet:

- Sesame seeds: 4 g net carbs = 7 g total carbs
- Pumpkin seeds: 2 g net carbs = 4 g total carbs
- Flax seeds: 0 g net carbs = 8 g total carbs
- Chia seeds: 2 g net carbs = 4 g total carbs
- Walnuts: 2 g net carbs = 4 g total carbs
- Pistachios: 5 g net carbs = 8 g total carbs
- Pecans: 1 g net carbs = 4 g total carbs
- Macadamia nuts: 2 g net carbs = 4 g total carbs
- Cashews: 8 g net carbs = 9 g total carbs
- Brazil nuts: 1 g net carbs = 3 g total carbs
- Almonds: 3 g net carbs = 6 g total carbs

Alternative Flours: Most wheat flours have a high carb count which makes them an enemy of the keto diet. The good news is that there are plenty of alternatives; here are some of them:

- Coconut flour
- Almond flour
- Pork rind dust
- Lupin flour
- Oat fiber

- Psyllium husk powder
- Flaxseed meal
- Chia flour

Don't Eat Too Much of These Foods

As you know, the keto diet is all about restricting your carbohydrate intake. To keep you in ketosis, keep these foods to a minimum:

- Baked goods
- Gluten-free baked goods
- Crackers and chips
- Sugar
- Syrup
- Honey
- Juices
- Sweetened yogurt
- Starchy vegetables
- High sugar fruits
- Grains

High Sugar Fruits: All fruits are healthy, but not when you're on the keto diet because some of them contain more sugar than others. These include:

- Pear: 1 medium pear contains 21 g net carbs = 27 g total carbs
- Mango: 1 cup contains 22 g net carbs and 25 g total carbs
- Dates: 2 large dates contain 32 g net carbs = 36 g total carbs
- Raisins: 28 g contains 21 g net carbs – 22 g total carbs
- Banana: 1 medium banana contains 24 g of net carbs = 27 g total carbs

Starchy Vegetables: Again, all vegetables are healthy, but not when you're on the keto diet because some of them contain more starch than others which can up your carb intake for the day. So, you can either avoid them all together or eat them in very limited amounts.

- Beets: 1 cup of cooked beets contains 14 g net carbs = 17 g total carbs
- Sweet potato: 1 medium sweet potato contains 20 g net carbs = 24 g total carbs
- Potato: 1 medium potato contains 33 g net carbs = 37 g total carbs
- Corn: 1 cup of corn contains 32 g net carbs = 36 g total carbs

Benefits of the Keto Diet

The obvious benefits of the ketogenic diet are weight loss. However, research suggests there are several other advantages, these include the following:

Hunger no More: One of the main reasons people don't like dieting is because they feel so hungry all the time. But this isn't the case when you're on a low-carb diet. When you eat more fat and protein, you stay full for longer which means you also eat less calories which is a win-win because it helps speed up the weight loss process. Also, once the body becomes accustomed to getting its energy from fat, it reduces cravings and reduces appetite so you're less likely to desire the sugary foods that were responsible for your weight gain in the first place.

Kills Candida: If you're prone to thrush outbreaks, you can say goodbye to them while you're on the keto diet.

Because you'll have reduced blood sugar levels, you'll have less glucose released from your urine. Bacteria feeds off glucose which creates the right environment for bacterial and yeast infections. Also, you'll be consuming more saturated fatty acids through foods such as coconut oil; a fatty acid called lauric acid contains antimicrobial properties which helps kill the germs associated with candida albican.

Clears up Acne: Acne has a number of different causes, but one of them is blood sugar and diet. Eating a high carbohydrate diet combined with processed foods causes extreme highs and lows in blood sugar, it also changes the balance of gut bacteria, both of which have a negative effect on skin health. A 2012 study reported in the National Library of Medicine found that participants suffering from acne on a ketogenic diet experienced improved symptom.

Reduced Risk of Cancer: Although experts agree there needs to be more research in this area, a 2018 study found that because the ketogenic diet reduces the risk of insulin complications, it also lowers the risk of cancer because research suggests that insulin complications are linked to some cancers.

Increased Mental Focus: A better memory, improved focus, and mental clarity are all benefits of the ketogenic diet due to an increase of healthy fats containing omega-3 fatty acids. Omega-3 fatty acids are found in oily fish such as mackerel, tuna and salmon and they are foods known to improve learning ability and mood because omega-3 fatty acids increase DHA levels which make up approximately one third of the brain.

Increased Weight Loss: One of the fastest ways to lose weight is to cut out carbohydrates. Studies have found that people on low-carb diets lose weight faster than those on low-fat diets even while restricting calories. Low-carb diets drain the body of excess water which lowers insulin levels and accelerates weight loss in the first two weeks.

A Flatter Stomach: Not all fat is created equal, and some fat is more stubborn than others. Additionally, the location of the fat determines the extent of the health risks. Fat around the stomach is called, 'visceral' fat and it's most common in men. This type of fat is affectionately known as a 'beer belly.' As funny as it might look, a beer belly is extremely dangerous and is associated with insulin resistance and inflammation. A low-carb diet attacks fat around the stomach quickly.

A Drop in Triglycerides: Too many fat particles in the bloodstream increase the risk of heart disease. People who don't do much exercise and eat a lot of carbs have high triglycerides, but this can be reduced on a low carbohydrate diet.

More Good Cholesterol: The body needs good cholesterol to protect it against heart disease, and contrary to popular belief, one of the best ways to do this is to eat a lot of fat.

A Drop in Blood Sugar and Insulin: A low-carb diet significantly reduces blood sugar and insulin levels. One study found that 95% of participants lowered or eliminated their medication within six months of starting the diet.

Reduces the Risk of Metabolic Syndrome: All the symptoms associated with metabolic syndrome were almost eliminated during a study reported in the Nutrition and Metabolism Journal. People with metabolic syndrome are more likely to suffer from diabetes and heart disease. Its symptoms include:

Low cholesterol

High triglycerides

High fasting blood sugar levels

High blood pressure

Treats Brain Disorders: One study found that 16% of epileptic children stopped having seizures while on the keto diet. The breakthrough led to experts using the keto diet to treat conditions such as Parkinson's and Alzheimer's disease.

Increased Energy: If you're tired of being on a perpetual energy roller coaster, the keto diet will stabilize your energy levels and prevent those mid-day slumps. When blood sugar levels are under control, your body will reward you with a constant supply of energy throughout the day.

Improved Sleep: Do you suffer from sleep problems? The ketogenic diet is the answer. You'll stop experiencing spikes in hormones such as melatonin, serotonin, and cortisol, all of which play an important role in sleep. Once these hormones are balanced, you'll have a good night's sleep every night.

Hormone Balancing: The keto diet is great for managing menopause symptoms such as brain fog and hot flashes. It's also good for treating menstrual issues and conditions such as polycystic ovary syndrome.

Reduced Inflammation: A combination of low-sugar and anti-inflammatory fats contribute to reduced inflammation levels in the body. High inflammatory markers are known to cause conditions such as arthritis, cardiovascular disease, and diabetes.

Air Fryer: Why it Works and Why it's an Amazing Find For Those on the Keto Diet

There are so many food choices with a keto diet that creativity is a must, and one way to achieve this is with an air fryer. The simplicity of its use and the variety of foods you can cook in it make dieting less stressful and more enjoyable. So, if you're ready to get more acquainted with the air fryer, keep reading.

What is an Air Fryer? Air fryers are the healthier alternative to deep fryers. They allow you to cook foods with little oil and get a similar texture and taste as fried foods. There are several functions on an air fryer that allow you to cook a wide variety of foods including vegetables, meats, and eggs.

How it Works: Air fryers use convection heat to push hot air around the machine to cook the food. The ingredients are made crispy by a process called the Maillard reaction which causes a crispy outer coating on the food. Most air fryers come with baskets or trays to allow for free-flowing air. Additionally, depending on the make, some air fryers have built in paddles that stir the food automatically while it's cooking so that you don't need to turn the food manually.

Air Fryer and Keto: As you've read, the keto diet consists of very high-fat and low-carb foods and it's important that their compounds are preserved during the cooking process. Also, the diet requires the consumption of a lot of meat which are difficult to cook without adding extra fats and grease. The air fryer enables you to cook with little to no oil which preserves the nutrients and makes for all round healthier meals.

The Deep-Frying Difference: Deep frying has gained a bad reputation over the years; however, it is especially disadvantageous for keto dieters because of the need to eat more healthy fats when on this diet. On a keto diet you need to get about 70% of your calories from fats. Bad fats are found in vegetable oils typically used for deep frying and they can clog your arteries, cause weight gain and increase your risk of heart disease. On the other hand, good fats lower cholesterol levels, decrease the risk of stroke, heart disease, and lower blood pressure. Additionally, heating cooking oil increases inflammatory compounds which are then soaked up by the foods which increases your risk of inflammation in the body. Since the air fryer requires less oil (one to two tablespoons per recipe), there is less risk of developing chronic disease. Finally, deep frying increases the amount of calories you eat per day because fried foods absorb fat and lose water which increases calorie count.

Advantages of the Air Fryer

While you can't cook everything in an air fryer, there are many benefits to using one for food preparation. Here are some of them:

Healthier: The most important benefit of using an air fryer is that it's healthier. You don't use much oil and any oil that is used drains away and is not absorbed by the food which means you eat less calories and fats.

Speed: You'll notice that a lot of the recipes in this book take less than 30 minutes to make and that includes meat, chicken, and fish dishes. That's because the heat and the fan action are so intense it speeds up the cooking process.

Safer: Deep fat frying can cause severe burns. With an air fryer, you don't need to worry about oil splashing everywhere or the food burning because once the timer ends, the machine shuts off.

Versatile: You can cook a lot of different recipes in an air fryer including steaks, vegetables, and baked goods. The added benefit is that they taste even better than when cooked in a traditional deep fryer.

Less Messy: You don't use a lot of oil with an air fryer which makes the cooking process less messy and the mess you do make, is easier to clean.

Less Wasteful: No matter what you're deep frying, it requires a lot of oil, although you can reuse the oil a couple of times, you've eventually got to get rid of it. You only need to use one to two teaspoons of oil with an air fryer, and as mentioned, you get the same results as the deep fryer.

Crispier Food: You get the true experience of eating fried foods with an air fryer. The difference is that it's healthier and tastes better. Everyone loves fried chicken, and French fries but not the health risks. The air fryer creates the same texture as deep-fried foods.

Air Fryer Keto Tips

As you've read, the air fryer will take your keto diet recipe making to the next level. But you can improve your experience by applying the following tips:

Keep an Eye on Less Weighty Foods

One of the components of an air fryer is a strong fan attached to its top, this can cause foods that don't hold much weight to blow around and get trapped in the heating element and burn. You can avoid this by holding the items down with a heat-safe trivet.

Don't Set it and Forget it

There is no one rule fits all when it comes to air frying so it's best to keep checking your food while it's cooking to ensure that you don't overcook or undercook it. This is even more important if you're cooking fish or poultry. Using a thermometer will help you determine whether the food is cooked properly.

Move Food Around

Shaking the basket or turning the food over will ensure that everything is evenly cooked. If not, you're likely to have part crispy and part soggy food items.

The Size of Your Vegetables

When it comes to air fryers, size matters. If you cut your vegetables too small, there's a chance they'll slip through the basket and burn on the coil. To prevent this, cut your vegetables so they're at least an inch in size.

Dry Foods and Spices

Let's say you season some broccoli and put them in the air fryer expecting some tasty florets. Once they're done, you can forget about seasoned broccoli because the fan will blow off all the seasoning. To keep the flavor stuck to your dry foods, spray them lightly with cooking oil before seasoning them.

Too Much Food in the Basket

If necessary, cook your foods in batches to avoid overfilling. It might take you a little longer to get your meals ready but at least the food will be cooked properly. The air fryer needs space so that air can circulate through the foods. Each air fryer basket will have a 'max fill' line on it, don't go past this.

Use the Right Oil

If you don't want dry food, stick to peanut, grapeseed, avocado, or extra light olive oil. A lot of oils have a low smoke point so even at a low temperature, they'll burn. The oils mentioned can withstand the heat and will give you the crispy texture you desire.

Preheat Your Air Fryer

Air fryers don't take long to warm up, but you want to make sure it's warm before you put your food in the basket, or it won't cook properly. All air fryers are different, your manual will tell you how long it takes to warm up your air fryer.

Read the Manual

Speaking of manuals, read every page of the manual before using your air fryer. Although it's boring to read, the manual will tell you everything you need to know about your air fryer to ensure you maximize its potential.

Chapter 2: Fast and Simple Recipes For Everyday Use

These recipes come in handy when you've got the munchies and you're looking for a quick fix to satisfy those hunger pangs. You won't be disappointed with the selection of recipes in this chapter.

Garlic and Lemon Shrimp

Nutrition: Calories: 190, Protein: 16 g, Fats: 12 g, Carbs: 2 g, Fiber: 1 g

Total Time: 10 minutes

Servings: 2

Ingredients:

- 8 oz (227 g) of deveined and shelled shrimp
- The juice of 1 medium lemon
- The zest of 1 medium lemon
- 2 tbsp of unsalted melted butter
- ½ tsp of old bay seasoning
- ½ tsp of minced garlic

Instructions:

1. Add all the ingredients to a large bowl and toss to coat the shrimp.
2. Transfer the shrimp mixture into a 9-inch baking pan.
3. Set the air fryer to 400° F (200° C).
4. Put the baking pan in the air fryer and cook for 6 minutes.
5. The shrimp will turn bright pink in color when cooked, and it should have an inside temperature of 120° F (50°C).
6. Remove from the air fryer and serve.

Pigs in a Blanket

Nutrition: Calories: 405, Protein: 17 g, Fats: 32 g, Carbs: 2 g, Fiber: 1 g

Total Time: 17 minutes

Servings: 2 servings

Ingredients:

- 2 oz (57 g) of beef smoked sausages
- 4 oz (113 g) of Mozzarella cheese
- ½ tsp of sesame seeds
- 1 oz (28 g) of full fat cream cheese
- 2 tbsp of blanched finely ground almond flour

Instructions:

1. In a large microwavable bowl, combine the Mozzarella, almond flour, and cream cheese. Heat for 45 seconds.
2. Remove the bowl from the microwave, whisk to combine, form a dough ball and slice it in half.
3. Flatten the dough balls to form a rectangle.
4. Lay a sausage in the middle of the dough, wrap and seal the edges.
5. Sprinkle the sesame seeds over the top.
6. Set the air fryer to 400° F (200°C).
7. Place the wrapped sausages in the air fryer and cook for 7 minutes.
8. Once they turn golden brown in color and the inside temperature is between 155-165° F (70°C), remove them from the air fryer and serve.

Crispy Fish Sticks

Nutrition: Calories: 205, Protein: 24 g, Fats: 10 g, Carbs: 1 g, Fiber: 1 g

Total Time: 25 minutes

Servings: 4

Ingredients:

- 1 oz (28 g) of finely ground pork rinds
- 1 pound (454 g) of cod fillets cut into ¾ inch strips
- 1 large egg
- 1 tbsp of coconut oil
- ½ tsp of Old Bay seasoning
- 1 oz (28 g) of blanched finely ground almond flour

Instructions:

1. In a large bowl, add the pork rinds, almond flour, coconut oil, and the Old Bay seasoning. Toss to combine.
2. Whisk the egg in a medium sized bowl.
3. Dip the fish sticks in the egg and then into the seasoning mixture.
4. Set the air fryer to 390° F (200°C).
5. Arrange the fish sticks in the air fryer and cook for 10 minutes.
6. Once the fish sticks turn golden brown in color and the inside temperature is 145° F (63°C), remove from the air fryer and serve.

Buffalo Chicken Wings

Nutrition: Calories: 750, Protein: 34 g, Fats: 64 g, Carbs: 1 g, Fiber: 1 g

Total Time: 35 minutes

Servings: 4

Ingredients:

- 2 pounds (907 g) of chicken wings
- 1 tsp of minced garlic
- 2 tbsp of apple cider vinegar
- 4 tbsp of unsalted butter
- 2 oz (71 g) of Buffalo hot sauce
- 2 oz (71 g) of avocado oil
- Avocado oil spray
- Salt and black pepper to taste
- 1 tsp of smoked paprika
- 2 tbsp of baking powder

Instructions:

1. In a large bowl, add the chicken wings, smoked paprika, baking powder and salt and pepper. Toss to combine and coat the chicken wings.
2. Spray the chicken wings with avocado oil.
3. Set the air fryer to 400° F (200°C).
4. Arrange the chicken wings in the air fryer and cook for 20 minutes.
5. Turn the chicken wings over after 10 minutes.

6. In a small saucepan, add the garlic, vinegar, butter, hot sauce, and avocado oil, heat over a low temperature and stir to combine.

7. The chicken is cooked once the inside temperature is 165° F (74 °C).

8. Once the chicken is cooked, remove them from the air fryer, coat with the buffalo sauce and serve.

Cheesy Bacon Rolls

Nutrition: Calories: 208, Protein: 6 g, Fats: 18 g, Carbs: 3 g, Fiber: 14 g

Total Time: 30 minutes

Servings: 4

Ingredients:

- 12 slices of bacon
- 6 large eggs
- 4 oz (113 g) of mild salsa
- 8 oz (228 g) of sharp Cheddar cheese, shredded
- ½ a medium green bell pepper seeded and chopped
- ½ oz (14 g) of chopped onion
- 2 tbsp of unsalted butter

Instructions:

1. Spoon the butter into a frying pan and melt over a low temperature.

2. Cook the peppers and onions for around 3 minutes.

3. Add the eggs, scramble them and remove them from the stove.

4. Arrange the bacon strips on a chopping board.

5. Spoon 3 tablespoons of the egg mixture onto the edge of the bacon strip.

6. Top with a 1 tablespoon of cheese, roll tightly and secure with a toothpick.

7. Set the air fryer to 350° F (177°C).

8. Arrange the rolls in the air fryer and cook for 15 minutes.

9. Turn the rolls over halfway through.

10. The bacon will become crispy and turn golden brown, and the inside temperature will be 150° F (66°C) when cooked.

11. Remove the rolls from the air fryer and serve with the salsa.

Spinach Bacon and Egg Muffins

Nutrition: Calories: 180, Protein: 11 g, Fats: 14 g, Carbs: 2 g, Fiber: 1 g

Total Time: 20 minutes

Servings: 6

Ingredients:

- 2 oz (57 g) of shredded Cheddar cheese
- 4 strips of cooked bacon, crumbled
- 1 oz (28 g) of chopped spinach
- ¼ tsp of ground black pepper
- ½ tsp of salt
- 2 oz (57 g) of heavy whipping cream
- 6 large eggs

Instructions:

1. In a large bowl, add the eggs, heavy whipping cream, salt and pepper and whisk to combine.

2. Divide the bacon and spinach in a six-cup silicone muffin holder.

3. Spoon the egg mixture into the muffin cups halfway.

4. Sprinkle cheese over the top.

5. Set the air fryer to 300° F (150°C).

6. Put the muffin holder in the air fryer for 14 minutes.

7. The inside temperature for the bacon will be 150° F (65°C) when cooked.

8. Once the eggs are firm and the cheese brown, remove from the air fryer and serve.

Savory Bagels

Nutrition: Calories: 224, Protein: 12g, Fats: 19g, Carbs: 2g, Fiber: 2g

Total Time: 30 Minutes

Servings: 6

Ingredients:

- 7 oz (198 g) of Mozzarella cheese
- 1 large egg, whisked
- 2 tbsp of unsalted butter
- 1 tsp of everything bagel seasoning
- 1/8 tsp of fine sea salt
- 1 tbsp of baking powder
- 3 oz (95 g) of blanched almond flour
- 1 tbsp of apple cider vinegar
- Avocado oil

Instructions:

1. Make the dough by combining the butter and Mozzarella in a large microwave safe bowl. Heat for 1 to 2 minutes in 30 second increments until the cheese is fully melted.

2. Remove the bowl from the microwave and stir to combine.

3. Add the egg and stir to combine.

4. Add the vinegar and stir to combine.

5. Slowly add the flour while mixing with a handheld mixer.

6. Add the baking powder and salt and whisk until fully combined.

7. Knead the dough out on a sheet of parchment paper, put it in a bowl, cover with clean film and leave the dough in the fridge for an hour.

8. Set the air fryer to 350° F (176°C).

9. Spray a 9-inch round baking pan with avocado oil.

10. Divide the dough into six equal parts and roll into a log.

11. Mold the log into a circle to form a bagel shape.

12. Do the same with the rest of the dough.

13. Lightly spray the bagels with avocado oil, sprinkle the bagel seasoning over the top and arrange in the baking pan.

14. Put the baking pan in the air fryer and cook for 14 minutes.

15. Turn halfway and remove from the air fryer once the bagels turn golden brown in color.

Sausage Sandwich

Nutrition: Calories: 759, Protein: 41 g, Fats: 61 g, Carbs: 15 g, Fiber: 3 g

Total Time: 35 minutes

Servings: 4

Ingredients For the Dough:

- 1 large egg
- 3 oz (95 g) almond flour
- 2 oz (57 g) cream cheese
- 8 oz (228g) mozzarella cheese

Ingredients For the Filling:

- 4 tbsp of sugar-free maple syrup
- 4 large eggs
- 4 large, cooked sausage patties

Instructions:

1. Set the air fryer to 400° F (200°C).
2. Put the cream cheese and mozzarella cheese into a microwavable safe bowl and heat for 30 seconds at a time until melted.
3. Remove the cheese from the microwave, stir to combine and add the egg and almond flour and stir to combine to form a dough.
4. Place the dough between two sheets of parchment paper and roll the dough into a rectangle.
5. Use a biscuit cutter or a cup to cut the bread.
6. Cook the bread for 7 minutes and flip halfway through.
7. While the bread is cooking, cook the sausage and egg.
8. The bread is cooked when it's crispy and golden brown in color.
9. Once the bread is cooked, remove it from the air fryer and set it to one side.
10. The sausage is cooked once the inside temperature is 155 – 165° F (74°C).
11. Spread maple syrup over the bread, arrange the sausage and egg onto it and serve.

Crispy Cod

Nutrition: Calories: 405, Protein: 41 g, Fats: 25 g, Carbs: 5 g, Fiber: 2 g

Total Time: 20 minutes

Servings: 2

Ingredients:

- 1 pound (454g) of cod fillets
- 1 tsp of salt
- 2 oz (57 g) of unsalted butter
- 2 slices of lemon
- Avocado oil spray

Instructions:

1. Set the air fryer to 400° F (200°C).
2. In a large bowl, season the cod with salt.
3. Spray the cod with avocado oil.
4. Place the cod in the basket and put a piece of butter and a slice of lemon on each piece of cod and cook for 10 minutes.
5. The cod is cooked when it turns golden brown in color and the inside temperature is 145° F (63°C).
6. Once cooked, remove the cod from the air fryer and serve.

Crispy Onion Rings

Nutrition: Calories: 135, Protein: 8 g, Fats: 7 g, Carbs: 5 g, Fiber: 5 g
Sugar 2 g

Total Time: 26 minutes

Servings: 4

Ingredients:

- ½ tsp garlic powder
- ½ tsp paprika
- 3 tbsp of blanched almond flour
- 1 oz (28 g) of pork rinds
- 2 large eggs
- ¼ tsp of sea salt
- 3 tbsp of coconut flour
- 1 large onion sliced into ½ inch thick rings
- Avocado oil spray

Instructions:

1. Set the air fryer to 400° F (200°C).
2. Combine the sea salt and coconut flour in one small bowl.
3. Whisk the eggs in another small bowl.
4. Combine the garlic powder, paprika, almond flour, and pork rinds in another small bowl.
5. Dip an onion in the egg, then coconut flour, and then the pork rind mixture.
6. Repeat with all the onion rings.
7. Spray the onion rings with avocado oil.
8. Arrange the onion rings in the air fryer and cook for 16 minutes.
9. The onion rings are cooked when they turn golden brown in color.
10. Once cooked, remove the onion rings from the air fryer and serve.

Roast Boneless Turkey Breast

Nutrition: Calories: 105, Protein: 2 g, Fats: 7 g, Carbs: 6 g, Fiber: 5 g

Total Time: 15 minutes

Servings: 4

Ingredients:

- 2 pounds (907g) boneless turkey breast
- ½ tsp of black pepper
- 1 tsp of salt
- 4 tbsp of olive oil
- 3 tbsp of Herbes de Provence
- 3 tbsp of dried rosemary

Instructions:

1. Set the air fryer to 350° F (176°C).
2. Put the turkey breasts into a large bowl, combine the rest of the ingredients and work the ingredients into the turkey breast with your clean hands.
3. Put the turkey breast in the air fryer and cook for 15 minutes.
4. Remove the turkey from the air fry, baste in olive oil and cook for another 10 minutes.
5. The turkey is cooked when it turns golden brown in color and the inside temperature is 165° F (74°C).
6. Once the turkey is cooked, remove from the air fryer and serve.

Spinach Stuffed Tomatoes

Nutrition: Calories: 267, Protein: 11 g, Fats: 21 g, Carbs: 10 g, Fiber: 4 g, Sugar: 5 g

Total Time: 35 minutes

Servings: 4

Ingredients:

- 4 beefsteak ripe tomatoes
- 1 oz (43 g) of grated Parmesan cheese
- 3 tbsp of cream cheese
- 5 oz (142g) of garlic and herb Boursin cheese
- 10 oz (284g) of fresh spinach
- ½ tsp of Kosher salt
- ¾ tsp of ground black pepper

Instructions:

1. Set the air fryer to 350° F (176°C).
2. Slice the tops off the tomatoes and spoon out the insides.
3. Season the insides of the tomatoes with salt and pepper.
4. Lay paper towels down and place the tomatoes cut side down on the paper towels to drain any excess water.
5. In a medium sized bowl, add the spinach, cream cheese, Boursin cheese, ¼ cup of Parmesan cheese and salt and pepper and stir to combine.
6. Spoon the spinach mixture into the tomatoes.
7. Sprinkle the remaining Parmesan cheese on top of the tomatoes.
8. Put the tomatoes into the air fryer and cook for 15 minutes.
9. The tomatoes are cooked when they become soft.
10. Once cooked, remove the tomatoes from the air fryer and serve.

Scallops With Creamy Tomato Sauce

Nutrition: Calories: 359, Protein: 9 g, Fats: 33 g, Carbs: 6 g, Fiber: 0 g, Sugar: 1 g

Total Time: 15 minutes

Servings: 2

Ingredients:

- 8 jumbo sea scallops
- 12 oz (340g) of spinach
- Avocado cooking oil spray
- ½ tsp of black pepper
- ½ tsp of salt
- 1 tsp of finely chopped garlic
- 1 tbsp of fresh basil, chopped
- 1 tbsp of tomato paste
- 6 oz (177 g) of heavy whipping cream

Instructions:

1. Set the air fryer to 350° F (176°C).
2. Spray a baking dish with avocado oil and arrange the spinach on the bottom of the pan.
3. Spray the scallops and season with salt and pepper.
4. Arrange the scallops on top of the spinach.
5. Combine the garlic, basil, tomato paste, cream, salt and pepper and whisk.

6. Pour the sauce over the scallops.
7. Put the baking dish in the air fryer and cook for 10 minut
8. The scallop is cooked when it has an internal temperature of 125-130° F (54°C).
9. Remove the baking dish from the air fryer and serve.

Crunchy Fried Pickles

Nutrition: Calories: 105, Protein: 2 g, Fats: 7 g, Carbs: 6 g, Fiber: 5 g

Total Time: 15 minutes

Servings: 4

Ingredients:

- 2 tbsp of heavy whipping cream
- 8 dill pickle spears
- 1 egg
- ½ tsp of garlic powder
- ½ oz (15 g) of crushed pork rind crumbs
- 1 oz (28 g) of almond flour
- Salt and pepper to taste
- Low-carb spicy Cajun dipping sauce to serve

Instructions:

1. Set the air fryer to 350° F (176°C).
2. Add the heavy whipping cream and the egg in a shallow bowl and whisk to combine.
3. Put the pork rind crumbs into a bowl.
4. Tip the almond flour out onto a plate.
5. Add the garlic powder, and salt and pepper to the almond flour and toss to combine.
6. Roll the pickle spears in the flour.
7. Soak the pickle spears in the egg.
8. Roll the pickle spears in the pork rinds.
9. Put the coated pickle spears into the air fryer and cook for 15 minutes.
10. The pickle spears are cooked once they turn golden brown and crispy.
11. Once cooked, remove the pickle spears from the air fryer and serve with a spicy Cajun dipping sauce.

Parmesan Flavored Chicken Tenders

Nutrition: Calories: 239, Protein: 29 g, Fats: 9 g, Carbs: 13 g, Fiber: 0 g

Total Time: 25 minutes

Servings: 4

Ingredients:

- 1 pound (454 g) skinless, boneless chicken cut into strips
- 1 tsp of Italian seasoning
- 2 oz (71 g) of almond flour
- 1 egg
- 1 oz (40 g) of breadcrumbs
- 1 oz (40 g) of grated Parmesan cheese
- Salt and pepper to taste
- Avocado cooking oil

Low-carb, sugar-free barbeque sauce

air fryer to 400° F (200°C).

e bread crumbs, whisked egg, and flour in three
rate shallow bowls.

d the salt, pepper, Italian seasoning, and Parmesan cheese
to the breadcrumbs and stir to combine.

4. Dip the chicken strips into the flour.

5. Dip the chicken strips into the egg.

6. Dip the chicken strips into the breadcrumbs.

7. Spray the chicken tenders with avocado oil and place them
into the air fryer.

8. Cook the chicken tenders for 8 minutes.

9. Flip the chicken tenders and cook them for a further 8
minutes.

10. The chicken tenders are cooked when they have an internal
temperature of 165° F (74°C) and they're crispy and brown on
the outside.

11. Once cooked, remove the chicken tenders from the air fryer
and serve with barbeque sauce.

Chapter 3: Breakfast Recipes

As the saying goes, "Start as you mean to go on." Start your day with a healthy breakfast and you're most likely to eat a healthy lunch and too. These recipes are quick and easy to make whether it's just for you, or your whole family.

Egg Cheese and Spinach Omelette

Nutrition: Calories: 368, Protein: 20g, Fats: 28g, Carbs: 2g, Fiber: 1g

Total Time: 17 Minutes

Servings: 2

Ingredients:

- 4 large eggs
- 1 oz (50 g) of mild cheddar cheese, shredded
- 2 tbsp of salted melted butter
- 2 tbsp of yellow onion, peeled and chopped
- 1 oz (45 g) of fresh spinach, chopped
- ¼ tsp of salt

Instructions:

1. Whisk the eggs in a round 12 cm baking dish.
2. Add the cheddar, butter, onion, spinach and salt. Stir to combine.
3. Set the air fryer temperature to 320° F (160°) .
4. Put the dish into the air fryer basket and cook for 12 minutes.
5. Once the omelette is light brown in color, it's ready to serve.

Tomato Egg & Spinach

Nutrition: Calories: 146, Protein: 14g, Fats: 8g, Carbs: 1g, Fiber: 0g

Total Time: 25 minutes

Servings: 4

Ingredients:

- 17 oz (485 g) of liquid egg whites
- ½ oz (15 g) of fresh spinach leaves
- ½ a medium Roma tomato cored and diced
- ¼ tsp of onion powder
- ¼ tsp of salt
- Cooking spray
- 3 tbsp of melted salted butter

Instructions:

1. Combine the egg whites, onion powder, butter and salt in a large bowl.
2. Add the spinach and tomato and stir to combine.
3. Grease four 8cm ramekins with cooking spray and pour the mixture into them.
4. Set the air the air fryer temperature to 302° F (150°C).
5. Place the ramekins into the air fryer and cook for 15 minutes.
6. Once the eggs are firm in the middle, they are ready to serve.

Pepper and Ham Omelette

Nutrition: Calories: 476, Protein: 41 g, Fats: 32 g, Carbs: 3 g, Fiber: 1 g

Total Time: 13 minutes

Servings: 1

Ingredients:

- 2 large eggs
- 1 oz (30 g) of cheddar cheese, shredded
- 2 tbsp of spring onions, diced
- 1 oz (30 g) of red and green peppers, diced
- 1.2 oz (35 g) of ham, diced
- 1/8 tsp of ground black pepper
- ¼ tsp of fine sea salt
- 2 fl oz (60 ml) of unflavored, unsweetened almond milk
- Cooking oil
- Optional: 3-4 cherry tomatoes sliced in half and 3 sticks of green onion, chopped

Instructions:

1. Grease a 6cm by 12 cm cake pan with cooking oil.
2. Combine the eggs, almond milk, pepper and salt in a small bowl.
3. Add the spring onions, ham, and diced peppers and stir to combine.
4. Pour the ingredients into the pan.
5. Top with cheese.
6. Set the air fryer to 400° F (200°C).
7. Put the pan in the air fryer and set the timer for 8 minutes.
8. The ham is cooked when the inside temperature reaches 145° F (63°C).
9. Once cooked, place the omelette on a plate and garnish with cherry tomatoes and onions if desired.

Peppers With Sausage

Nutrition: Calories: 489, Protein: 23 g, Fats: 35 g, Carbs: 13 g, Fiber: 4 g

Total Time: 30 minutes

Servings: 4

Ingredients:

- 4 oz (115 g) of full fat sour cream
- 8 tbsp of pepper jack cheese, shredded
- 4 large poblano peppers
- 2.1 oz (60 g) of canned diced green chilies and diced tomatoes
- 4 oz (115 g) of full fat softened cream cheese
- 4 large eggs
- 8.1 oz (230 g) of spicy pork sausage meat

Instructions:

1. Heat a medium skillet over medium temperature.
2. Crumble the sausage into the skillet and cook until it turns completely brown.
3. Use a slotted spoon to scoop the sausage out of the pan and transfer into a large bowl.
4. Pour the fat from the saucepan into a separate bowl (dispose of in a way that's most convenient for you).
5. Put the skillet back onto the stove and scramble the eggs until

they become firm.

6. Pour the cream cheese over the sausage and stir to combine.

7. Add the chilies and diced tomatoes and stir to combine.

8. Add the eggs and stir to combine.

9. Remove the seeds and the white membrane from the poblano peppers by making a 8-10cm slit through the top of the peppers with a small knife.

10. Spoon the sausage mixture into each of the peppers.

11. Sprinkle each pepper with 2 tablespoons of pepper jack cheese.

12. Heat the air fryer to 356° F (180°C).

13. Place the peppers into the air fryer and cook for 15 minutes.

14. The sausage is cooked when the inside temperature is 155-165° F (74°C).

15. Once the cheese is light brown and the peppers are soft, remove them from the air fryer and arrange onto plates.

16. Top the peppers with a dollop of sour cream and serve.

Sausage Egg Cup

Nutrition: Calories: 267, Protein: 14 g, Fats: 21 g, Carbs: 1 g, Fiber: 0 g

Total Time: 25 minutes

Servings: 6

Ingredients:

- 6 large eggs
- 12 oz (340 g) of pork meat sausage
- ½ tsp of crushed red pepper flakes
- ¼ tsp of ground black pepper
- ½ tsp of salt
- Cooking oil

Instructions:

1. Grease six 8cm ramekins with cooking oil.

2. Arrange the sausage in the ramekins by pressing the meat into the bottom and up the sides, it should be about 1cm thick.

3. Crack one egg into each ramekin.

4. Sprinkle with red pepper flakes, and salt and pepper.

5. Set the air fryer to 350° F (177°C).

6. Arrange the ramekins in the air fryer and cook for 15 minutes.

7. The sausage is cooked when the inside temperature is 155-165° F (74°C).

8. Once the eggs are firm, remove from the air fryer and serve.

Egg Pepperoni

Nutrition: Calories: 241, Protein: 19 g, Fats: 15 g, Carbs: 4 g, Fiber: 0 g

Total Time: 15 minutes

Servings: 2

Ingredients:

- 7 slices of chopped pepperoni
- 1 large whisked egg
- 3 oz (8 g) of Mozzarella cheese, shredded
- ¼ tsp of salt
- ¼ tsp of garlic powder
- ¼ tsp of dried parsley

- ¼ tsp of dried oregano

Instructions:

1. Tip the Mozzarella cheese onto the bottom of an ungreased 12 cm round non-stick baking dish.

2. Spread the pepperoni over the cheese.

3. Pour the whisked egg over the top.

4. Sprinkle the spices over the top.

5. Set the air fryer to 329° F (165°C).

6. Place the dish into the air fryer and cook for 10 minutes.

7. When the cheese has browned and the egg has set, remove from the air fryer and serve.

Almond and Pecan Granola

Nutrition: Calories: 617, Protein: 11 g, Fats: 55 g, Carbs: 21 g, Fiber: 11 g, Sugar: 10.2 g

Total Time: 15 minutes

Servings: 6

Ingredients:

- 5 oz (140 g) of almond slivers
- 7 oz (220 g) of chopped pecans
- 1 tsp of ground cinnamon
- 2 tbsp of unsalted butter
- 1/8 oz (5 g) of granulated sweetener
- 1/8 oz (5 g) of low-carb sugar-free chocolate chips
- 1 oz (40 g) of golden flaxseeds
- 1 oz (40 g) of sunflower seeds
- 3 oz (90 g) of unsweetened coconut flakes

Instructions:

1. Add all the ingredients to a large bowl and stir to combine.

2. Transfer the mixture into a round baking dish.

3. Put the dish into the air fryer.

4. Set the air fryer to 320° F (160°C).

5. Cook for five minutes.

6. Leave to cool down before serving

Breakfast Lemon Cake

Nutrition: Calories: 204, Protein: 6 g, Fats: 18 g, Carbs: 17 g, Fiber: 2 g, Sugar: 8 g

Total Time: 15 minutes

Servings: 6

Ingredients:

- 1 tsp of poppy seeds
- The juice of 1 medium lemon
- 1 tbsp of lemon zest
- 1 tsp of vanilla extract
- 2 large eggs
- 2 oz (60ml) of unsweetened almond milk
- 2 oz (55 g) of melted unsalted butter
- ½ tsp of baking powder
- 1/3 oz (10 g) of powdered sweetener
- 3 oz (95 g) of blanched finely ground almond flour

Instructions:

1. Add the eggs, almond milk, vanilla, butter, baking powder, sweetener, and almond flour into a large bowl and stir to combine.
2. Add the lemon juice and stir to combine.
3. Add the lemon zest and stir to combine.
4. Add the poppy seeds and stir to combine.
5. Transfer the batter into a 12cm non-stick round cake pan.
6. Place the cake pan into the air fryer.
7. Set the air fryer to 300° F (148°C).
8. Cook for 14 minutes.
9. Once cooked, stick a tooth pick through the center and if it comes out clean, the cake is ready.
10. Leave the cake to cool down to room temperature before serving.

Ham and Avocado Delight

Nutrition: Calories: 307, Protein: 14 g, Fats: 24 g, Carbs: 3 g, Fiber: 7g

Total Time: 15 minutes

Servings: 2

Ingredients:

- 7/8 oz (25 g) of Cheddar cheese, shredded
- ¼ tsp of ground black pepper
- ½ tsp of fine sea salt
- 2 tbsp of chopped spring onions
- 2 large eggs
- 2 slices of thin ham
- 1 large Hass avocado, sliced in half and pitted

Instructions:

1. Push the ham into the hole in each avocado slice.
2. Crack an egg on top of the ham.
3. Add a dash of spring onions.
4. Sprinkle salt and pepper over the top.
5. Set the air fryer to 300° F (158°C).
6. Put the avocado halves into the air fryer and cook for 10 minutes.
7. The ham is cooked when the inside temperature is 145° F (63°C).
8. Once cooked, top with cheese, cook for another 30 seconds and serve.

Egg and Ham Delight

Nutrition: Calories: 281, Protein: 18 g, Fats: 18 g, Carbs: 6 g, Fiber: 2 g

Total Time: 25 minutes

Servings: 4

Ingredients:

- 4 large eggs whisks
- 3 oz (100 g) of shredded mild Cheddar cheese
- ½ tsp of salt
- ½ oz (15 g) of white onion peeled and chopped
- 3 oz (85 g) of cooked ham, chopped

- 1 tbsp of coconut oil
- 4 green peppers, seeded

Instructions:

1. Add salt to the whisked eggs and put to one side.
2. Drizzle coconut oil over the peppers.
3. Add the onions and ham into each pepper.
4. Pour the eggs into each pepper.
5. Add Cheddar cheese to each pepper.
6. Arrange the peppers in the air fryer.
7. Set the air fryer to 300° F (148°C).
8. The ham is cooked when the inside temperature is 145° F (63°C).
9. Cook for 15 minutes, the eggs will be firm and the peppers tender when ready.

Golden Muffins

Nutrition: Calories: 160 g, Protein: 5 g, Fats: 14 g, Carbs: 20 g, Fiber: 2 g

Total Time: 20 minutes

Servings: 6

Ingredients:

- 1 tsp of ground allspice
- 2 tsp of baking powder
- 1 large egg
- 2 tbsp of melted butter
- 1/8 oz (5 g) of granulated sweetener
- Cooking spray
- 3 oz (95 g) of blanched finely ground almond flour

Instructions:

1. Add all the ingredients to a large bowl and whisk to combine.
2. Grease a six muffin cup holder with cooking spray.
3. Pour the batter into the muffin cup holder.
4. Set the air fryer to 300° F (148°C).
5. Place the muffin holder into the air fryer and cook for 15 minutes.
6. Serve warm.

Cheddar Cheese Egg

Nutrition: Calories: 359, Protein: 20g, Fats: 27 g, Carbs: 1 g, Fiber: 0 g

Total Time: 15 minutes

Servings: 2

Ingredients:

- 1 oz (50 g) of sharp Cheddar cheese, shredded
- 2 tbsp of unsalted butter
- 4 large eggs

Instructions:

1. Whisk the eggs in a large baking dish.
2. Set the air fryer to 400° F (205°C).
3. Place the baking dish inside the air fryer.
4. Set the timer for 10 minutes.
5. After 5 minutes stir the eggs, add the cheese and butter and cook for 3 minutes.

6. Stir again and cook for another two minutes.

7. Once cooked, remove from the air fryer and serve.

Chocolate Chip Muffin

Nutrition: Calories: 329, Protein: 10 g, Fats: 29 g, Carbs: 20 g, Fiber: 8 g, Sugar: 14 g

Total Time: 20 minutes

Servings: 6

Ingredients:

- 3 oz (85 g) of low-carb chocolate chips
- 1 tbsp of baking powder
- 2 large eggs
- 4 tbsp of salted melted butter
- ½ oz (15 g) of granulated sweetener
- 5 oz (145 g) of blanched finely ground almond flour

Instructions:

1. Add all the ingredients into a large bowl and stir to combine.

2. Grease a six-cup silicone muffin tray.

3. Spoon the batter into the muffin cups.

4. Set the air fryer to 300° F (148°C).

5. Place the muffin tray into the air fryer.

6. Cook for 15 minutes.

7. Once the muffins are golden brown, remove them from the air fryer.

8. Leave the muffins to cool down for 15 minutes before serving.

Hash Brown Cauliflower

Nutrition: Calories: 153, Protein: 10 g, Fats: 9 g, Carbs: 3 g, Fiber: 2 g

Total Time: 20 minutes

Servings: 4

Ingredients:

- 3 oz (100 g) of sharp Cheddar cheese, shredded
- 1 large egg
- 1 bag of steamer cauliflower (12 oz or 340 g)

Instructions:

1. Cook the bag of cauliflower in the microwave according to the instructions on the packet.

2. Once cooked, removed the cauliflower bag from the microwave.

3. Pour the cauliflower into a tea towel and squeeze out the excess water.

4. Transfer the cauliflower into a bowl, add the egg and cheese.

5. Line a sheet of parchment paper in your air fryer basket.

6. Spoon ¼ of the hash brown mixture into the air fryer basket and shape into a hash brown. Do this until you've made 4 hash browns.

7. Set the air fryer to 400° F (204°C).

8. Cook for 12 minutes and flip the hash browns after 6 minutes.

9. Once the hash browns are golden brown in color, they are ready to serve.

Broccoli Frittata

Nutrition: Calories: 16, Protein: 10 g, Fats: 11 g, Carbs: 2 g, Fiber: 1 g,

Sugar: 5.7 g

Total Time: 27 minutes

Servings: 4

Ingredients:

- 1 oz (30 g) of chopped green pepper
- 1 oz (20 g) of chopped yellow pepper
- 1 oz (50 g) of chopped broccoli
- 1 oz (50 g) of chopped onion
- 2 oz (60 g) of heavy whipped cream
- 6 large eggs

Instructions:

1. Combine the eggs, heavy whipping cream, pepper, onion, and broccoli and whisk together thoroughly.

2. Pour the mixture into a 12cm round baking dish.

3. Place the baking dish into the air fryer.

4. Set the temperature to 300° F (148°C).

5. Cook for 12 minutes.

6. The eggs will be firm once cooked.

Blueberry Muffins

Nutrition: Calories: 269, Protein: 8 g, Fats: 24 g, Carbs: 20 g, Fiber: 3 g

Total Time: 20 minutes

Servings: 6

Ingredients:

- 1 oz (45 g) of fresh chopped blueberries
- 2 tbsp of baking powder
- 2 large eggs
- 4 tbsp of salted melted butter
- 1/3 oz (10 g) of granulated sweetener
- 4 oz (115 g) of blanched finely ground almond flour
- Cooking spray

Instructions:

1. Add all the ingredients to a large bowl and stir to combine.

2. Grease a 6 muffin tray with cooking spray.

3. Spoon the mixture into the muffin tray.

4. Set the air fryer to 300° F (148°C).

5. Cook the muffins for 15 minutes.

6. Once the muffins are golden brown in color, remove them from the air fryer.

7. Leave the muffins to cool down for 15 minutes before serving.

Turkey Sausage

Nutrition: Calories: 170, Protein: 16 g, Fats: 11 g, Carbs: 1 g, Fiber: 0 g

Total Time: 35 minutes

Servings: 6 (2 patties per person)

Ingredients:

- 24 oz (680 g) of lean ground turkey
- ½ tsp of cayenne pepper
- ½ tsp of paprika
- 1 tsp of dried thyme
- 1 tsp of Creole seasoning

- 1 tsp of Tabasco sauce
- ¼ grated onion
- 3 cloves of finely chopped garlic

Instructions:

1. Put all the ingredients into a large bowl, and combine with your hands.
2. Shape the mixture into 12 patties about ½ an inch thick.
3. Arrange the patties into the air fryer.
4. Set the air fryer to 370° F (188°C).
5. Cook the patties for 20 minutes turning over at 10 minutes.
6. The patties are cooked when the inside temperature is 165° F (74°C).
7. Once cooked, remove from the air fryer and serve.

Mushroom Frittata

Nutrition: Calories: 360, Protein: 25 g, Fats: 25 g, Carbs: 10 g, Fiber: 2 g

Total Time: 35 minutes

Servings: 2

Ingredients:

- 2 oz (58 g) of Parmesan cheese
- 6 large eggs
- ¼ tsp of freshly ground black pepper
- ½ tsp of salt
- ½ oz (13 g) of finely chopped onion
- 1 oz (50 g) sliced brown mushrooms
- 10 oz (284 g) of finely chopped broccoli florets
- 1 tbsp of olive oil

Instructions:

1. Add the mushrooms, broccoli, onion, olive oil, salt and pepper to an 8 inch non-stick baking pan and toss to combine.
2. Set the air fryer to 400° F (204°C).
3. Place the baking pan into the air fryer and cook for 5 minutes until the vegetables become soft. Remove the baking pan from the air fryer.
4. Add the eggs and the Parmesan cheese to a medium sized bowl and whisk to combine.
5. Pour the eggs over the cooked vegetables and put the baking pan back into the air fryer for another 15 minutes until the eggs are firm.

Tomato and Mushroom Medley

Nutrition: Calories: 255, Protein: 11 g, Fats: 20 g, Carbs: 7 g, Fiber: 3 g

Total Time: 30 minutes

Servings: 2

Ingredients:

- 2 large eggs
- 1 tbsp of freshly chopped parsley
- 2 tbsp of Pecorino Romano cheese
- 2 Roma tomatoes cut in half
- 2 Portobello mushrooms, gills and stems removed
- ¼ tsp of dried thyme
- 2 cloves of minced garlic
- 1 tbsp of olive oil

- Salt and pepper to season

Instructions:

1. In a small bowl, add the thyme, garlic, and olive oil and whisk to combine.
2. Brush the mixture over the tomatoes and mushrooms and season with salt and pepper.
3. Set the air fryer to 400° F (204°C).
4. Place the mushrooms and tomatoes in the air fryer cut side up.
5. Crack an egg into the middle of each mushroom.
6. Sprinkle cheese over the top of the mushrooms.
7. Cook for 15 minutes until the eggs are firm.
8. Remove the mushrooms and tomatoes from the air fryer.
9. Leave the tomatoes to cool down before slicing them and scattering them on top of the eggs.
10. Garnish with parsley and serve.

Pork Sausage Egg With Mustard Sauce

Nutrition: Calories: 340, Protein: 22 g, Fats: 28 g, Carbs: 1 g, Fiber: 0 g

Total Time: 35 minutes

Servings: 6

Ingredients:

- 1 oz (28g) of crushed pork rinds
- 2 tbsp olive oil
- 1 large egg
- 6 hardboiled eggs
- 1 pound (454 g) of pork sausage

Smoky Mustard Sauce

- 1 tsp of chipotle hot sauce
- 1 tbsp of Dijon mustard
- 2 tbsp of sour cream
- 2 oz (58 g) of mayonnaise

Instructions:

1. Form the sausage meat into 6 patties
2. Place 1 boiled egg in the middle of each patty and wrap the patty around the egg so that it's completely covered.
3. Whisk the egg in a small bowl.
4. Put the pork rinds into another small bowl.
5. Dip one wrapped sausage egg into the egg and then into the pork rinds until evenly coated. Repeat with all patties.
6. Set the air fryer to 390° F (200°C).
7. Place the sausage eggs into the air fryer, spray with olive oil and cook for 15 minutes.
8. Prepare the sauce by combining the hot sauce, Dijon mustard, sour cream and mayonnaise in a small bowl. Whisk to combine and serve with the sausage eggs.
9. The sausage is cooked when the inside temperature is 165° F (74°C).
10. Once cooked, remove from the air fryer and serve.

Egg Bacon Cheese & Avocado

Nutrition: Calories: 512, Protein: 27 g, Fats: 38 g, Carbs: 5 g, Fiber: 3 g

Total Time: 35 minutes

Servings: 4

Ingredients:

- 6 large eggs
- 12 slices of bacon, cooked and crumbled
- 2 tbsp of cheese
- 8 tbsp of sour cream, full-fat
- 1 medium avocado, peeled, pitted and sliced into 8 pieces
- 3 oz (100g) of chopped cauliflower
- 2 oz (60g) of heavy whipping cream

Instructions:

1. Add the cream and eggs to a large mixing bowl and whisk until combined.
2. Pour the egg mixture into a 4-cup round baking dish.
3. Arrange the cauliflower over the top.
4. Top with cheese.
5. Set the air fryer to 320° F (160°C).
6. Place the baking dish in the air fryer and cook for 20 minutes.
7. The bacon is cooked once the inside temperature is 150° F (66°C).
8. Once the eggs are firm and the cheese has browned, serve with avocado slices, bacon, and sour cream.

Aromatic Cake

Nutrition: Calories: 153, Protein: 5 g, Fats: 13 g, Carbs: 11 g, Fiber: 2 g

Total Time: 20 minutes

Servings: 4

Ingredients:

- 1.6 oz (48g) of blanched finely ground almond flour
- ½ tsp of ground cinnamon
- ½ tsp of vanilla extract
- ½ tsp of unflavored gelatine
- 1 large egg
- 2 tbsp of softened unsalted butter
- ½ tsp of baking powder
- 1 oz (45 g) of powdered erythritol

Instructions:

1. Combine the almond flour, baking powder, cinnamon, butter, vanilla, gelatine, egg, and erythritol in a large bowl until a batter is formed.
2. Pour the batter into a 6-inch round baking pan.
3. Set the air fryer to 300° F (148°C).
4. Put the baking pan into the air fryer and cook for 7 minutes.
5. Check the cake is cooked by sticking a toothpick in the middle of it. If it comes out clean, it's ready.

Cheese and Bacon Flatbread

Nutrition: Calories: 361, Protein: 26 g, Fats: 24 g, Carbs: 5 g, Fiber: 0 g

Total Time: 15 minutes

Servings: 2

Ingredients:

- 8 oz (223 g) Mozzarella cheese, shredded

- 1 oz (28 g) of cream cheese, crumbled
- 1 large egg
- ¼ tsp of chopped jalapenos
- 4 slices of chopped bacon, cooked
- ¼ tsp of salt

Instructions:

1. Pour the Mozzarella out into a 6-inch round baking dish.
2. Top with the cream cheese pieces.
3. Top with the cooked bacon.
4. Add the jalapenos.
5. Whisk the egg with salt and pour it over the top.
6. Set the air fryer to 330° F (165°C).
7. Put the baking dish into the air fryer and cook for 10 minutes.
8. The bacon is cooked when the inside temperature is 150° F (65°C).
9. When the egg is set and the cheese is browned, it's ready to serve.

Avocado and Sausage

Nutrition: Calories: 276, Protein: 22 g, Fats: 17 g, Carbs: 1 g, Fiber: 3 g

Total Time: 20 minutes

Servings: 4

Ingredients:

- 1 pound (454 g) of ground turkey breakfast sausage
- 2 tbsp of mayonnaise
- 1 medium avocado, pitted, peeled, and sliced
- 1 oz (50 g) green peppers, seeded and chopped
- ¼ tsp of ground black pepper
- ½ tsp of salt

Instructions:

1. Add all the ingredients into a large bowl and combine with your hands.
2. Form four meat patties and arrange them in the air fryer.
3. Set the air fryer to 370° F (188°C).
4. Cook the patties for 15 minutes and turn half way.
5. The sausage is cooked when the inside temperature is 155 – 165° F (74°C).
6. Once the patties are cooked, serve them with the sliced avocados.

Cheesy Sausage Meatballs

Nutrition: Calories: 288, Protein: 11 g, Fats: 24 g, Carbs: 1 g, Fiber: 0 g

Total Time: 25 minutes

Servings: 6 (18 meatballs, 3 per person)

Ingredients:

- 1 large egg
- 1 pound (454 g) of ground pork breakfast sausage
- 1 oz (28 g) of soft cream cheese
- 4 oz (113 g) of sharp Cheddar cheese
- ¼ tsp of salt
- ¼ tsp of black pepper

Instructions:

1. Put all the ingredients in a large bowl, use your hands to combine.

2. Form the mixture into 18 meatballs.

3. Set the air fryer to 300°F (148° C).

4. Arrange the meatballs in the air fryer and cook for 15 minutes.

5. The meatballs are cooked when the inside temperature is between 155 – 165° F (74°C).

6. Once the meatballs are crispy and brown, they're ready to serve.

Chapter 4: Appetizers and Snacks

Snacking is every dieter's downfall; the good news is that there are plenty of healthy snacking options, and you'll find them right here in this chapter as well as some scrumptious appetizers that make the perfect, 'just before dinner treat.'

Crunchy Spinach Chips

Nutrition: Calories: 128, Protein: 2 g, Fats: 12 g, Carbs: 2 g, Fiber: 1 g

Total Time: 30 minutes

Servings: 3 servings

Ingredients For Spinach Chips:

- 3 oz (85 g) of fresh spinach leaves
- 1 tsp of garlic powder
- ½ tsp of cayenne pepper
- 1 tsp of sea salt
- 1 tbsp of extra virgin olive oil

Ingredients for Chili Yogurt Dip

- ½ tsp of chili powder
- 2 tbsp of mayonnaise
- 2 oz (57 g) of yogurt

Instructions:

1. Tip the spinach leaves into a bowl, add the seasonings and olive oil and toss to combine.
2. Set the air fryer to 350° F (176° C).
3. Cook the spinach for 10 minutes, shaking the basket twice during the cooking process.
4. While the spinach is cooking, make the dip by adding all the ingredients to a small bowl and whisk to combine.
5. Once the edges are brown, remove from the air fryer and serve with the dip.

Parmesan Bell Pepper

Nutrition: Calories: 163, Protein: 6 g, Fats: 11 g, Carbs: 9 g, Fiber: 1 g

Total Time: 20 minutes

Servings: 4

Ingredients:

- 1 large egg
- 1 oz (43 g) of grated Parmesan cheese
- 2 tbsp of olive oil
- 8 bell peppers, seeded and sliced into ¼ inch strips
- ½ tsp of crushed red pepper flakes
- 1 tsp of sea salt

Instructions:

1. Add the egg, Parmesan cheese, olive oil, red pepper flakes, and salt to a medium sized bowl and stir to combine.
2. Add the bell peppers and toss to combine.
3. Set the air fryer to 390° F (198°C).
4. Cook the bell peppers for 10 minutes, shaking the basket after 5 minutes.
5. Once the bell peppers are soft but tender, remove and serve.

Tomato Cheesy Flavored Chips

Nutrition: Calories: 130, Protein: 5 g, Fats: 10 g, Carbs: 5 g, Fiber: 1 g

Total Time: 20 minutes

Servings: 4

Ingredients:

- 1 oz (45 g) of grated Parmesan cheese
- 1 tsp of Italian mixed seasoning
- Salt and white pepper to taste
- 2 tbsp of olive oil
- Cooking spray
- 4 sliced Roma tomatoes

Instructions:

1. Grease the air fryer basket with cooking spray.
2. Add all the ingredients to a bowl and toss to combine.
3. Set the air fryer to 350° F (177°C).
4. Arrange the tomatoes in the air fryer and cook for 10 minutes.
5. Shake the basket after five minutes.
6. Remove from the air fryer and serve.

Bacon and Zucchini Cheese Cake

Nutrition: Calories: 311, Protein: 18 g, Fats: 25 g, Carbs: 5 g, Fiber: 2 g

Total Time: 30 minutes

Servings: 4

Ingredients:

- 3 oz (85 g) grated Cotija cheese
- 2 medium eggs, lightly whisked
- ¾ oz (25 g) of coconut flour
- ¾ oz (25 g) of almond meal
- 7.9 oz (225 g) of chopped bacon
- 1 tsp of Mexican oregano
- ½ tsp of freshly cracked black pepper
- 1 zucchini grated and trimmed
- ½ tbsp of finely chopped grated basil
- 1.2 oz (33 g) of finely chopped scallions
- 1/3 tsp of baking powder
- 1/3 tsp of fine sea salt
- 1.2 oz (33 g) of grated Swiss cheese
- Mayonnaise to serve
- Ketchup to serve
- Cooking spray

Instructions:

1. Combine all the ingredients (except the Cotjia cheese) in a large bowl and stir to combine.
2. Use your hands to roll the mixture into balls and then flatten slightly to get the shape of cup-cakes.

3. Spray the cakes with cooking spray.

4. Set the air fryer to 305° F (152°C).

5. Cook the cakes for 15 minutes.

6. The bacon is cooked when the inside temperature is 150° F (66°C).

7. Serve warm with Cotija cheese, mayonnaise and ketchup.

Crispy Cauliflower

Nutrition: Calories: 160, Protein: 3 g, Fats: 14 g, Carbs: 5 g, Fiber: 3 g

Total Time: 20 minutes

Servings: 2

Ingredients:

- 6 oz (198 g) cauliflower florets
- 1 tsp of paprika
- 1 tsp of rosemary
- 1 tsp of sage
- 1 tsp of thyme
- 1 tsp of garlic powder
- 1 tsp of onion powder
- 2 tbsp of sesame oil

Instructions:

1. Put all the ingredients into a large bowl and toss until the cauliflower is properly coated.

2. Set the air fryer to 400° F (204° C) degrees.

3. Add the cauliflower to the basket, cook for 12 minutes and shake half way through.

4. Once the cauliflower is crispy, it's ready to serve.

Chicken Nuggets With Cheese

Nutrition: Calories: 268, Protein: 2 g, Fats: 18 g, Carbs: 4 g, Fiber: 1 g

Total Time: 20 minutes

Servings: 6

Ingredients:

- 1 lb (454 g) of chicken breasts sliced into tenders
- 2 oz (57 g) sugar free barbecue sauce
- 2 oz (57 g) of mayo
- 1 oz (43 g) of freshly grated Parmesan cheese
- 1 large egg, whisked
- ¾ oz (24 g) of almond meal
- ½ tsp of cayenne pepper
- Salt and black pepper for seasoning

Instructions:

1. Season the chicken tenders with cayenne pepper, black pepper, and salt.

2. Dip the chicken tenders into the almond meal.

3. Dip the chicken tenders into the whisked egg.

4. Coat the chicken tenders with Parmesan cheese.

5. Set the air fryer to 360° F (182°C).

6. Arrange the chicken tenders in the air fryer and cook for 10 minutes.

7. Turn the chicken tenders after five minutes.

8. Combine the mayonnaise and barbecue sauce in a small bowl.

9. The chicken is cooked when the inside temperature is 165° F (74°C).

10. Once the chicken tenders are cooked, serve with the sauce.

Cheese Burgers on a Stick

Nutrition: Calories: 469, Protein: 3 g, Fats: 30 g, Carbs: 4 g, Fiber: 1 g

Total Time: 30 minutes

Servings: 4

Ingredients:

- 1 lb (454 g) of ground beef
- 12 cubes of Cheddar cheese
- 12 cherry tomatoes
- Salt and pepper for seasoning
- ½ tsp of cumin
- 1 tsp of minced garlic
- 2 tbsp of minced scallions
- 1 tbsp of Dijon mustard
- Skewers

Instructions:

1. Add the ground beef, scallions, garlic, mustard, cumin, salt and pepper to a large bowl and use your hands to combine.

2. Form 12 round meatballs.

3. Set the air fryer to 375° F (190°C).

4. Cook for 15 minutes until the meatballs are golden brown in color.

5. The meatballs are cooked when the inside temperature is 160° F (71°C).

6. Thread one meatball, cheese, and cherry tomato on a stick. Repeat three times to make 4 skewers and serve.

Pork Meatballs

Nutrition: Calories: 275, Protein: 3 g, Fats: 18 g, Carbs: 2 g, Fiber: 1 g

Total Time: 20 minutes

Servings: 6 servings (12 meatballs, 2 per person)

Ingredients:

- 24 oz (680 g) of ground pork
- 2 chopped yellow onions
- 5 cloves of minced garlic
- 2 tbsp of grated Brie cheese
- 2 tsp of mustard
- 1 tsp of cayenne pepper
- Sea salt and ground black pepper for seasoning

Instructions:

1. Add all the ingredients to a large bowl and use your hands to combine.

2. Form the mixture into 12 meatballs.

3. Set the air fryer to 375° F (190°C).

4. Place the meatballs in the air fryer and cook for 15 minutes.

5. The meatballs are ready to serve once they turn golden brown in color and the inside temperature is 145° F (63°C).

Roasted Zucchini

Nutrition: Calories: 270, Protein: 3 g, Fats: 15 g, Carbs: 5 g, Fiber: 1 g

Total Time: 30 minutes

Servings: 6

Ingredients:

- 24 oz (680 g) of zucchini, peeled and sliced into ½ inch chunks
- 2 tbsp of finely chopped sage
- 1 pinch of salt and pepper
- 2 tbsp of coconut oil
- The zest of 1 small lemon
- 1/8 tsp of ground allspice

Instructions:

1. Put all the ingredients into a large bowl and toss to combine.
2. Set the air fryer to 350° F (177°C).
3. Arrange the zucchinis in the air fryer and cook for 10 minutes.
4. Turn the temperature up to 400° F (204°C), shake the basket and cook for another 10 minutes.
5. Once the zucchinis become golden brown in color, they are ready to serve.

French Fry Styled Broccoli With Spicy Dip

Nutrition: Calories: 219, Protein: 5 g, Fats: 19 g, Carbs: 9 g, Fiber: 3 g

Total Time: 25 minutes

Servings: 4

Ingredients For the Broccoli Fries:

- 12 oz (340 g) of broccoli
- 4 tbsp of grated parmesan cheese
- 2 tbsp of sesame oil
- Sea salt and ground black pepper to taste
- ½ tsp of cayenne pepper
- 1 tsp of garlic powder
- ½ tsp of onion powder
- Cooking oil

Ingredients For the Spicy Dip

- 1 tsp of keto hot sauce
- ¼ tsp of Dijon mustard
- 2 oz (57 g) of Greek yogurt
- 2 oz (57 g) of mayonnaise

Instructions:

1. Boil a large saucepan of water.
2. Blanch the broccoli for 4 minutes.
3. Grease the air fryer basket with cooking oil.
4. Drain the broccoli, add to a dry them with kitchen paper.
5. Add the broccoli, cheese and seasonings to a large bowl and toss to combine.
6. Set the air fryer to 350° F (176°C).
7. Put the broccoli in the air fryer and cook for 10 minutes. Shake the basket halfway through.
8. Make the sauce by adding the ingredients to a small bowl and whisk to combine.
9. Once the broccoli French fries are cooked, serve with the dip.

Succulent Seasoned Eggplant

Nutrition: Calories: 241, Protein: 4 g, Fats: 21 g, Carbs: 9 g, Fiber: 5 g

Total Time: 40 minutes

Servings: 4

Ingredients:

- 1 eggplant, peeled and thinly sliced
- ½ tsp of black pepper
- ½ tsp of salt
- ½ tsp of dried dill weed
- 1 tsp of garlic powder
- 4 oz (113 g) of water
- 2 oz (57 g) of olive oil
- 1 oz (48 g) of almond meal

Instructions:

1. Lay the eggplant slices on a tea towel, salt them and let them sit for 30 minutes.
2. Rinse the eggplant under cold water and squeeze out the excess water.
3. Put all the ingredients into a bowl and toss to combine.
4. Set the air fryer to 390° F (198° C) and cook for 15 minutes.
5. Once the eggplant has turned golden brown in color, they are ready to serve.

Golden Brussels Sprouts

Nutrition: Calories: 174, Protein: 3 g, Fats: 3 g, Carbs: 9 g, Fiber: 4 g

Total Time: 30 minutes

Servings: 4

Ingredients:

- 1 lb (454 g) of Brussels sprouts, yellow leaves and ends removed and sliced in half
- 1 handful of fresh chopped parsley
- 1 tsp of fennel seeds
- 1 tbsp of toasted sesame oil
- Salt and pepper to taste

Instructions:

1. Combine all the ingredients (except the parsley) in a Ziploc bag and shake to combine.
2. Set the air fryer to 380° F (193°C).
3. Arrange the Brussels sprouts in the air fryer and cook for 15 minutes.
4. Shake the basket half way through.
5. Once the Brussels sprouts turn golden brown in color, they are ready.
6. Garnish with fresh parsley and serve.

Kale Chips

Nutrition: Calories: 11, Protein: 1 g, Fats: 1 g, Carbs: 2 g, Fiber: 1 g

Total Time: 15 minutes

Servings: 6 servings

Ingredients:

- 2 large bunches of kale
- 1/8 tsp of ground black pepper

- 1/8 tsp of sea salt
- ¼ tsp of onion powder
- ¼ tsp of garlic powder
- ½ tsp of dried parsley
- ½ tsp of dried dill weed
- ½ tsp of dried chives
- Cooking oil

Instructions:

1. Wash the kale and pat them completely dry with paper towels.
2. Cut out the stems.
3. Add the kale and the seasoning to a large bowl and toss to combine.
4. Spray the air fryer basket with cooking oil.
5. Set the air fryer to 360° F (182°C).
6. Place the kale in the air fryer in a single layer and cook for 10 minutes, shaking halfway through.
7. Layer a baking tray with baking paper, arrange the kale onto the baking tray and leave to cool down completely.
8. Sprinkle with salt before serving.

Pork Belly Vinegar Flavored Chips

Nutrition: Calories: 240, Protein: 13 g, Fats: 21 g, Carbs: 0 g, Fiber: 0 g

Total Time: 45 minutes

Servings: 4

Ingredients:

- 1 lb (454 g) of pork belly
- 4 oz (113 g) of apple cider vinegar
- Fine sea salt
- Cooking oil

Ingredients For Serving

- Pico de gallo
- Guacamole

Instructions:

1. Cut the pork belly into 1/8-inch-thick strips and lay them in a shallow dish.
2. Pour the vinegar, sea salt over the top and put the dish in the fridge for 30 minutes.
3. Spray the air fryer basket with cooking oil.
4. Set the air fryer to 400° F (204° C).
5. Arrange the pork belly in the air fryer and cook for 15 minutes.
6. Flip the pork bellies halfway through.
7. Once the pork belly has turned crispy and brown, and the inside temperature is 145° F, remove from the air fryer and serve with guacamole and pico de gallo.

Crunchy Pepperoni Chips

Nutrition: Calories: 69, Protein: 3 g, Fats: 5 g, Carbs: 0 g, Fiber: 0 g

Total Time: 15 minutes

Servings: 2

Ingredients:

- 14 slices of pepperoni
- Cooking spray

Instructions:

1. Spray the air fryer basket with cooking spray.
2. Set the air fryer to 350° F (177°C).
3. Cook the pepperoni for 8 minutes until they have turned brown in color and crispy.
4. Remove the pepperoni from the air fryer and leave to cool down for 5 minutes before serving.

Cheesy Pickle Spear

Nutrition: Calories: 160, Protein: 7 g, Fats: 11 g, Carbs: 8 g, Fiber: 2 g

Total Time: 45 minutes

Servings: 4 servings

Ingredients:

- 4 dill pickle spears cut into half lengthwise
- 2 tbsp of dry ranch seasoning
- 1 oz (43 g) of grated Parmesan cheese
- 1 oz (48 g) blanched finely ground almond flour

Instructions:

1. Soak up the pickle juice from the spears by wrapping them in kitchen towel for 30 minutes.
2. In a medium sized bowl, add the ranch seasoning, Parmesan cheese, and flour and stir to combine.
3. Coat the pickle spears in the mixture.
4. Set the air fryer to 400° F (204°C).
5. Arrange the pickle spears in the air fryer and cook for 10 minutes.
6. Turn the pickle spears over halfway through cooking.
7. Once the pickle spears turn golden brown in color, remove from the air fryer and serve.

Avocado French Fries

Nutrition: Calories: 282, Protein: 15 g, Fats: 22 g, Carbs: 2 g, Fiber: 7 g,

Total Time: 25 minutes

Servings:

Ingredients:

- 3 firm avocados, cut in half, pitted and peeled
- 1 handful of chopped fresh cilantro
- 2 large eggs
- ½ tsp of onion powder
- ½ tsp of garlic powder
- 1 tsp of paprika
- 1 tsp of chili powder
- 2 tsp of ground cumin
- 2 tsp of ground black pepper
- 2 tsp of fine sea salt
- 2 oz (68 g) of pork dust
- Avocado oil spray

Ingredients For Serving

- Salsa

Instructions:

1. Slice the avocados into French fry shapes.
2. Add the seasonings, pork dust, and salt and pepper in a medium sized bowl and toss to combine.

3. Whisk the eggs in a small bowl.

4. Dip the avocado fries into the eggs, and then the seasoning mix.

5. Spray the fries with avocado oil.

6. Spray the air fryer basket with avocado oil.

7. Set the air fryer to 400° F (204° C).

8. Arrange the avocado fries in the air fryer and cook for 15 minutes.

9. Flip the avocado fries halfway through.

10. When the avocado fries are golden brown in color and crispy, they are ready.

11. Top with fresh cilantro and serve with salsa.

Zucchini Cheesy Fries

Nutrition: Calories: 124, Protein: 5 g, Fats: 10 g, Carbs: 4 g, Fiber: 1 g

Total Time: 2 hours 20 minutes

Servings: 6

Ingredients:

- 2 medium zucchinis
- 1 tsp of Italian seasoning
- 2.2 oz (62 g) grated Parmesan cheese
- 1 oz (50 g) of blanched finely ground almond flour
- 2 oz (80 g) of whipping cream
- ½ tsp of salt

Instructions:

1. Slice the ends of the zucchini, cut them into quarters and then into fries, 3-inch in length.

2. Remove the excess moisture by wrapping the zucchini in kitchen towels for 2 hours.

3. Pour the cream and salt into a medium sized bowl.

4. In another medium sized bowl, add the Italian seasoning, Parmesan cheese, and flour and toss to combine.

5. One by one, dip the zucchini fry into the cream, and then the dry ingredients.

6. Set the air fryer to 400° F (204°C).

7. Arrange the zucchini fries in the air fryer and cook for 10 minutes.

8. Turn the zucchini fries halfway through.

9. Once the zucchini fries are golden brown and crispy, they are ready to serve.

10. Lay a sheet of parchment paper on a baking tray, arrange the zucchini fries on the baking tray and leave to cool for 5 minutes before serving.

Crunchy Salami Cheese Roll-Ups

Nutrition: Calories: 269, Protein: 11 g, Fats: 22 g, Carbs: 2 g, Fiber: 0 g

Total Time: 5 minutes

Servings: 4 (16 roll-ups, 4 per person)

Ingredients:

- 14 oz (397 g) of Genoa salami deli slices
- 4 oz (113 g) of cream cheese

Instructions:

1. Spoon some cream cheese onto the edge of a slice of salami and roll. Put a toothpick in the middle to secure the salami in

place.

2. Repeat the process with the rest of the salami.

3. Arrange the salami roll-ups in a non-stick baking dish.

4. Set the air fryer to 350° F (177°C).

5. Put the baking dish into the air fryer and cook for 4 minutes.

6. Once the salami is crispy.

7. Remove the salami roll ups from the air fryer and leave to cool down for 5 minutes before serving.

Cauliflower Bacon Skewers

Nutrition: Calories: 69, Protein: 5 g, Fats: 5 g, Carbs: 2 g, Fiber: 1 g

Total Time: 25 minutes

Servings: 4

Ingredients:

- 4 slices of bacon cut into three pieces
- 4 oz (113 g) of cauliflower florets
- ¼ yellow medium onion sliced into 1-inch pieces
- ¼ tsp of salt
- 1 tsp garlic powder
- 1 tsp of olive oil
- Skewers

Instructions:

1. Thread 1 piece of bacon through a skewer.

2. Thread 2 pieces of onion on top.

3. Thread 1 piece of bacon on top.

4. Thread 2 pieces of cauliflower florets on top.

5. Thread 1 piece of bacon on top.

6. Repeat the process with 3 more skewers.

7. Drizzle olive oil over the skewers.

8. Sprinkle the skewers with garlic powder and salt.

9. Set the air fryer to 375° F (190°C).

10. Cook the skewers for 12 minutes.

11. Turn the skewers halfway through.

12. Once the bacon is crispy and golden brown in color and the inside temperature is 150° F (66° C) and the vegetables are tender, the skewers are ready to serve.

Cheesy Chicken and Pork

Nutrition: Calories: 395, Protein: 30 g, Fats: 27 g, Carbs: 2 g, Fiber: 1 g

Total Time: 10 minutes

Servings: 2

Ingredients:

- 1 oz (28 g) pork rinds
- 2.2 oz (62 g) full-fat sour cream
- 2.2 oz (62 g) guacamole
- 2.2 oz (62 g) sliced pickled jalapenos
- 4 oz (112 g) Monterey jack cheese, shredded
- 4 oz (112 g) cooked chicken, shredded

Instructions:

1. Arrange the pork rinds into a 6-inch round baking pan.

2. Top with the shredded chicken.

3. Top with the Monterey jack cheese.

4. Set the air fryer to 370° F (188°C).

5. Put the baking pan into the air fryer and cook for 5 minutes until the cheese has melted.

6. The chicken is cooked when the inside temperature is 165° F (74°C).

   Remove the baking pan from the air fryer, top with sour cream, guacamole, and jalapenos and serve.

Pork Rind Cheesy Tortillas

Nutrition: Calories: 145, Protein: 11 g, Fats: 10 g, Carbs: 1 g, Fiber: 0 g

Total Time: 15 minutes

Servings: 4

Ingredients

- 1 oz (28 g) of pork rinds
- 1 large egg
- 2 tbsp of full-fat cream cheese
- 2.2 oz (63 g) Mozzarella cheese, shredded
- Salsa for serving

Instructions:

1. Put the pork rinds into a food processor and pulse until they are finely ground.

2. Add the Mozzarella cheese, the cream cheese to a large microwaveable bowl and heat at 30 second increments until the cheese melts.

3. Remove the cheese from the microwave and stir to combine.

4. Add the egg and the pork rinds to the cheese and stir until a dough is formed.

5. Form the dough into four balls, place each ball between two sheets of parchment paper and roll into flat tortillas.

6. Set the air fryer to 400° F (204°C).

7. Arrange the tortillas into the air fryer and cook for 5 minutes.

8. Once the tortillas are crispy and golden brown in color, remove from the air fryer and serve with salsa.

Golden Egg Pork

Nutrition: Calories: 141, Protein: 10 g, Fats: 10 g, Carbs: 1 g, Fiber: 0 g

Total Time: 25 minutes

Servings: 4 (3 egg halves per person)

Ingredients:

- 6 large hardboiled eggs
- 1 large egg
- 1 oz (28 g) of finely crushed plain pork rinds
- ¼ tsp of ground black pepper
- ¼ tsp of salt
- Cooking spray
- 2 tbsp of mayonnaise

Instructions:

1. Slice the eggs in half and remove the yolks, put them into a separate bowl and move to one side.

2. Whisk the egg in a small bowl.

3. Put the pork rinds in a separate small bowl.

4. Dip the egg white into the egg.

5. Dip the egg into the pork rinds.

6. Spray the eggs with cooking spray.

7. Set the air fryer to 400° F (204°C).

8. Arrange the eggs in the air fryer and cook for 5 minutes.

9. Turn the eggs over halfway through.

10. Add the mayonnaise to the egg yolks, sprinkle with salt and pepper and stir to combine.

11. Once the eggs are golden, remove them from the air fryer.

12. Spoon the egg yolk mixture into the middle of the coated egg white and serve.

Chicken Wings and Eggs

Nutrition: Calories: 317, Protein: 24 g, Fats: 24 g, Carbs: 1 g, Fiber: 0 g

Total Time: 40 minutes

Servings: 4 (12 chicken wings, 3 per person)

Ingredients:

- 1 dozen chicken wings
- 2 tsp of berbere spice
- 1 tsp of fine sea salt
- 1 tbsp of coconut oil

Ingredients For Serving:

- ¼ tsp of dried chives
- 2 hard large hard-boiled eggs
- ½ tsp of fine sea salt

Instructions:

1. Put the chicken wings in a large bowl and coat with oil.

2. Add the salt and berbere seasoning and use your hands to work into the chicken.

3. Set the air fryer to 380° F (193°C).

4. Arrange the chicken in the air fryer and cook for 25 minutes.

5. Flip the chicken after 15 minutes.

6. Turn the temperature up to 400° F (204° C) and cook the chicken for another 6 minutes.

7. Slice the hard-boiled eggs in half and season with salt and dried chives.

8. Once the chicken is crispy and brown and the inside temperature is 165° F (74°C), serve with the seasoned eggs.

Cheesy Chicken Wings

Nutrition: Calories: 565, Protein: 42 g, Fats: 42 g, Carbs: 2 g, Fiber: 0 g

Total Time: 30 minutes

Servings: 4

Ingredients:

- 32 oz (907 g) of chicken wings
- 2.6 oz (75 g) grated Parmesan cheese
- 2 oz (54 g) dried parsley
- 1 tbsp of baking powder
- ½ tsp of garlic powder
- 1 tsp of pink Himalayan salt
- 4 tbsp of unsalted butter

Instructions:

1. In a large bowl, combine the chicken wings, baking powder,

salt, and garlic powder. Use your hands to work the
ingredients into the chicken.

2. Set the air fryer to 400° F (204°C).

3. Arrange the chicken wings in the air fryer and cook for 25
minutes.

4. Toss the chicken a few times while it's cooking.

5. In a small bowl, add the parsley, Parmesan, and butter and stir
to combine.

6. The chicken is cooked when the inside temperature is 165° F
(74°C).

7. Once the chicken is cooked, remove them from the air fryer,
coat with the butter mixture and serve.

When most people think about poultry, the first thing that comes to mind is chicken. But there are plenty of other delicious birds to add to the menu such as turkey, and duck. Here is a wonderful selection of savory poultry recipes to choose from.

BBQ Chicken Kebabs

Nutrition: Calories: 225, Protein: 25 g, Fats: 12 g, Carbs: 5 g, Fiber: 1 g

Total Time: 1 hour 25 minutes

Servings: 5

Ingredients:

- 1 lb (454 g) of chicken breasts cut into 1-inch cubes
- 5 grape tomatoes
- 2 tbsp of coconut aminos
- 1 tbsp of chicken seasoning
- 1 tsp of BBQ seasoning
- ½ a yellow pepper, diced
- ½ a green pepper, diced
- ½ a red pepper, diced
- ½ a zucchini, diced
- ½ a onion, diced
- Salt and ground black pepper to taste
- Cooking oil spray
- Skewers

Instructions:

1. In a large bowl, add the chicken, coconut aminos, chicken seasoning, BBQ seasoning, and salt and pepper. Use your hands to combine everything.
2. Cover the chicken with cling film and put it in the fridge to marinate for 1 hour.
3. Thread 1 piece of marinated chicken through a wooden skewer.
4. Thread a piece of onion, pepper, and zucchini.
5. Thread a piece of chicken.
6. Thread a piece of onion, pepper, and zucchini.
7. Thread a piece of chicken.
8. Thread a grape tomato.
9. Repeat this process with the remaining 4 skewers.
10. Spray the skewers with cooking oil.
11. Layer a grill rack with parchment paper.
12. Set the air fryer to 350° F (177°C).
13. Arrange the chicken skewers on the grill rack.
14. Cook for chicken kebabs for 10 minutes, flip and cook for another 10 minutes.
15. Once the chicken is golden brown and crispy and the inside temperature is 165° F (74°C), remove from the air fryer and serve.

Turkey Pot Pie

Nutrition: Calories: 359, Protein: 17 g, Fats: 32 g, Carbs: 5 g, Fiber: 2 g

Total Time: 50 minutes

Servings: 6

Ingredients:

- 1 recipe Fathead pizza dough
- 2 oz (65 g) of frozen baby peas
- 26 oz (732 g) cooked, turkey, chopped
- ½ tsp of xanthan gum
- 2 oz (57 g) of cream cheese
- 5 oz (160 g) heavy whipping cream
- 15 oz (420 g) of turkey broth
- 1 tsp of ground black pepper
- 1 tsp of sea salt
- 1 tsp of minced garlic
- 2 chopped celery stalks
- 2.6 oz (74 g) chopped mushrooms
- 2 chopped shallots
- 4 tbsp unsalted butter

Instructions:

1. Set the air fryer to 325° F (163°C).
2. Spoon the butter into a large saucepan and melt it over medium temperature.
3. Add the garlic, celery, mushrooms, shallots, salt and pepper, stir to combine and fry for 1 minute.
4. Add the xanthan gum, cream cheese, heavy cream and broth and stir to combine.
5. Reduce the temperature to low and let the ingredients simmer for 5 minutes stirring constantly.
6. Add the turkey and the peas and stir to combine.
7. Spoon the mixture into 6 ramekins.
8. Place the pizza dough between 2 sheets of parchment paper and roll it out.
9. Cut the dough to fit the ramekins.
10. Place the dough over the fillings and use a knife to slit the top so the crust can vent.
11. Put the ramekins into the air fryer and cook for 20 minutes.
12. The pie is cooked when the crusts turn golden brown in color and the inside temperature of the turkey is 165° F (74°C).
13. Remove the ramekins from the air fryer and serve.

Spicy Chicken

Nutrition: Calories: 366, Protein: 11 g, Fats: 9 g, Carbs: 33 g, Fiber: 1 g

Total Time: 30 minutes

Servings: 4

Ingredients:

- 8 oz (240 g) of minced chicken
- 1 tsp of salt
- ½ tbsp of chili sauce
- ½ tsp of fresh grated ginger
- 1 tbsp of coconut aminos
- ½ tsp of fresh minced basil

- 1 tbsp of ground black pepper
- 3 cloves of minced garlic
- 1.2 oz (35 g) of chopped scallions
- 1/3 tsp of paprika

Instructions:

1. Put all the ingredients in a large bowl and combine with your hands.
2. Form four patties.
3. Set the air fryer to 355° F (179°C).
4. Cook the patties for 18 minutes.
5. Once the patties are golden brown in color and the inside temperature is 165° F (74°C), remove from the air fryer and serve.

Bacon and Chicken With Tomato

Nutrition: Calories: 296, Protein: 34 g, Fats: 13 g, Carbs: 5 g, Fiber: 2 g

Total Time: 30 minutes

Servings: 4

Ingredients:

- 2 chopped slices of smoked bacon
- 4 chicken drumsticks with the skin on
- 1 thinly sliced small leek
- 12 oz (340 g) of crushed canned tomatoes
- 2 cloves of crushed garlic
- 2 tbsp of olive oil
- 1 tbsp of rice vinegar
- Salt and pepper to taste
- 1 tsp of herbs de Provence

Instructions:

1. Put all the ingredients in a large bowl and stir to combine.
2. Set the air fryer to 360° F (182°C).
3. Transfer the ingredients into a baking dish and then into the air fryer.
4. Cook for 10 minutes.
5. Stir the ingredients and cook for a further 15 minutes.
6. The chicken is cooked when the inside temperature is 165° F (74°C).
7. The bacon is cooked when the inside temperature is 150° F (66° C).
8. Remove from the air fryer and serve.

Sweet & Crisp Duck Legs

Nutrition: Calories: 481, Protein: 26 g, Fats: 26 g, Carbs: 39 g, Fiber: 0.4 g

Total Time: 25 minutes

Servings: 2

Ingredients For the Duck:

- 2 duck legs (20 oz or 567 g)
- Avocado oil spray
- Salt and pepper to taste

Ingredients For the Glaze

- ¼ tsp of crushed red pepper flakes
- ½ tsp of sugar-free ketchup

- 1 tbsp of freshly squeezed orange juice
- 1 tbsp of sugar-free barbeque sauce
- 2 oz (80 g) of orange marmalade

Instructions:

1. Set the air fryer to 400° F (204°C).
2. Spray the duck legs with avocado oil and season with salt and pepper.
3. Place the duck legs into the air fryer and cook for 15 minutes.
4. The duck is cooked when it has an internal temperature of 165° F (74° C) and its golden brown in color.
5. Once cooked, remove the duck from the air fryer and let it rest for 10 minutes.
6. To make the glaze, add the red pepper flakes, ketchup, orange juice, barbeque sauce, and orange marmalade to a small saucepan and whisk to combine.
7. Let the glaze simmer for 10 minutes over low temperature.
8. Once the glaze is cooked, brush it over the duck legs and serve.

Chicken and Bacon With Cheese

Nutrition: Calories: 612, Protein: 16 g, Fats: 44 g, Carbs: 38 g, Fiber: 1 g

Total Time: 1 hour

Servings: 2

Ingredients:

- 2 chicken fillets
- 4 rashers of smoked bacon
- 1 oz (45 g) of grated Parmesan cheese
- 4 oz (123 g) of coconut milk
- 1 tsp of mild curry powder
- 1 tsp of black mustard seeds
- 1 piece of ginger (2-inches), peeled and minced
- 1 clove of garlic, minced
- ¼ tsp of ground black pepper
- ½ tsp of coarse sea salt

Instructions:

1. Set the air fryer to 400° F (204°C).
2. Cook the bacon for 5 minutes and remove from the air fryer.
3. Combine the coconut milk, curry powder, mustard seeds, ginger, garlic, black pepper, salt and chicken fillets in a large bowl. Stir together thoroughly and put the bowl in the fridge to marinate for 30 minutes.
4. Tip the Parmesan cheese into a medium sized bowl.
5. Dip the marinated chicken into the Parmesan cheese.
6. Set the air fryer to 380° F (193°C).
7. Arrange the chicken in the air fryer and cook for 6 minutes.
8. The chicken is cooked when the inside temperature is 165° F (74°C).
9. The bacon is cooked when the inside temperature is 150° F (66°C).
10. Once the chicken in crispy and golden brown in color, remove from the air fryer and serve with the bacon.

Cheesy Vegetable Chicken

Nutrition: Calories: 361, Protein: 1 g, Fats: 29, Carbs: 23 g, Fiber: 1 g

Total Time: 45 minutes

Servings: 4

Ingredients:

- 10 oz (296 g) chicken, cooked and shredded
- 3 cloves of finely chopped garlic
- ½ a thinly sliced red onion
- 17 oz (480 g) of mixed vegetables
- 1/3 tsp of crushed red pepper flakes
- 1 tsp of sea salt
- 2.4 oz (68 g) of grated Fontina cheese
- ½ tsp of dried marjoram
- 3 whisked eggs
- Vegetable oil

Instructions:

1. Combine all the ingredients (except the cheese) in a large bowl.
2. Grease a baking dish with vegetable oil.
3. Transfer the ingredients into the baking dish.
4. Set the air fryer to 365° F (185° C).
5. Put the baking dish in the air fryer and cook for 25 minutes.
6. The chicken is cooked when the inside temperature is 150° F (66°C).
7. Once cooked, top with the Fontina cheese and serve.

Turkey Meatballs

Nutrition: Calories: 149, Protein: 28 g, Fats: 3 g, Carbs: 2 g, Fiber: 1 g

Total Time: 15 minutes

Servings: 6

Ingredients:

- 1 lbs (680 g) of ground turkey
- ½ oz (14 g) of chopped Italian parsley
- 1 red medium bell pepper
- 1 large egg
- ½ tsp of ground black pepper
- ½ tsp of salt

Instructions:

1. Set the air fryer to 400° F (204° C).
2. Combine the ground turkey, egg, Italian parsley, bell pepper, salt and pepper in a large bowl and use your hands to bind together.
3. Shape the mixture into meatballs and put them into the air fryer.
4. Cook the meatballs for 10 minutes.
5. The meatballs are cooked when they become crispy and golden brown in color, and the inside temperature is 165° F (74°C).
6. Remove the meatballs from the air fryer and serve.

Chicken Breast in White Wine

Nutrition: Calories: 471, Protein: 12 g, Fats: 28 g, Carbs: 31 g, Fiber: 0,

Total Time: 30 minutes

Servings: 1

Ingredients:

- 3 boneless, medium sized chicken breasts sliced into cubes
- 1/3 tsp of freshly cracked black pepper
- ½ tsp of minced thyme leaves
- 4 oz (118 g) dry white wine
- 3 finely chopped green garlic stalks
- 1 tbsp of sesame oil
- ½ tsp of sea salt flakes
- 2.8 oz (79 g) of coconut milk
- ½ tsp fresh grated ginger

Instructions:

1. Pour the sesame oil into a saucepan and heat over medium temperature.
2. Sauté the green garlic until it becomes fragrant.
3. Take the saucepan off the stove and add the white wine and coconut milk and stir to combine.
4. Add the ginger, sea salt, black pepper and thyme and stir to combine.
5. Transfer the mixture into a baking dish.
6. Add the chicken cubes and stir to combine.
7. Set the air fryer to 335° F (169°C).
8. Put the baking dish in the air fryer and cook for 30 minutes.
9. Stir after 15 minutes.
10. The chicken is cooked when the inside temperature is 165° F (74°C).
11. Once cooked, remove from the air fryer and serve.

Cauliflower Chicken

Nutrition: Calories: 234, Protein: 2 g, Fats: 12 g, Carbs: 9 g, Fiber: 2 g

Total Time: 15 minutes

Servings: 6 servings

Ingredients:

- 6 chicken drumsticks
- ½ tsp of sea salt
- 1 tsp of freshly cracked pink pepper corns
- 1 tsp of garlic powder
- ½ tsp of shallot powder
- 1/3 tsp of sweet paprika
- 1 tsp of berbere spice
- 1/3 tsp of porcini powder
- 2 tsp of mustard powder
- 1 heads of cauliflower broken into florets
- 2 sprigs of thyme
- 4 oz (115 g) fresh chives, chopped
- 2 handfuls of chopped fresh parsley

Instructions:

1. Add all the ingredients to a medium sized bowl and stir to combine.
2. Put the cauliflower into the seasoning and gently toss to combine.
3. Transfer the cauliflower to the air fryer basket.
4. Put the chicken drumsticks into the mixture and use your

hands to work the seasoning into the chicken.

5. Transfer the chicken drumsticks to the air fryer basket.
6. Set the air fryer to 355° F (179°C).
7. Cook the chicken and cauliflower for 30 minutes.
8. The chicken is cooked when the inside temperature is 165° F (74°C).
9. Once the chicken and the cauliflower are golden brown in color, remove from the air fryer and serve.

Chicken Burgers With Cheese

Nutrition: Calories: 234, Protein: 6 g, Fats: 12 g, Carbs: 12 g, Fiber: 1 g

Total Time: 25 minutes

Servings: 4

Ingredients:

- 1 lb (454 g) of ground chicken meat
- 1 oz (28 g) of grated Parmesan cheese
- 1 tsp of freshly cracked black pepper
- 1/3 tsp of crushed red pepper flakes
- 2 tsp of cumin powder
- 1 tsp of sea salt flakes
- 1/3 tsp of porcini powder
- ½ tsp of onion powder
- 2 tsp of dried parsley flakes
- 1/3 tsp of ancho chili powder
- 2 tsp of dried marjoram
- 1 tsp of dried basil

Instructions:

1. In a large bowl, combine all the ingredients and form into patties.
2. Sprinkle Parmesan cheese over the top of each patty.
3. Set the air fryer to 345° F (174°C).
4. Arrange the patties in the air fryer and cook for 15 minutes.
5. Turn the patties over halfway.
6. The chicken is cooked when the inside temperature is 165° F (74°C).
7. Once the cheese and the patties are golden brown in color, remove from the air fryer and serve.

Chinese Crispy BBQ Duck

Nutrition: Calories: 502, Protein: 42 g, Fats: 34 g, Carbs: 3 g, Fiber: 3 g

Total Time: 30 minutes

Servings: 2

Ingredients:

- 2 large duck breasts
- 1 tbsp of minced garlic
- 4 tbsp of honey
- 2 tbsp of five-star spice seasoning
- 6 tbsp of soy sauce
- 5 tbsp of oyster sauce

Instructions:

1. Set the air fryer to 300° F (149°C).
2. Pat the duck breast completely dry using a paper towel.

3. Score the skin of the duck breasts with a sharp knife in a criss cross pattern from top to bottom.
4. Combine 2 tablespoons of honey, garlic, 1 tablespoon of five-star spice seasoning, 4 tablespoons of soy sauce, and 5 tablespoons of oyster sauce in a container and whisk together thoroughly. Make sure the container is big enough to fit the two pieces of duck in it.
5. Put the duck breasts into the container with the skin facing upwards.
6. Put plastic wrap over the container, and poke holes in it for ventilation.
7. Add 1 tablespoon of five-star spice seasoning, 1 tablespoon of honey, and 3 tablespoons of warm water to a small bowl and whisk to combine.
8. Put the duck into a baking dish.
9. Put the baking dish into the air fryer and cook for 15 minutes.
10. Add the honey mixture and cook for another 10 minutes.
11. The duck is cooked when the inside temperature is 155° F (68°C) and it's crispy and golden brown in color.
12. Once cooked, remove the duck from the air fryer and serve.

Creamy Chicken

Nutrition: Calories: 362, Protein: 8 g, Fats: 27 g, Carbs: 17 g, Fiber: 1 g

Total Time: 1 hour 30 minutes

Servings: 4

Ingredients:

- 1 lb (454 g) of boneless, skinless chicken thighs cut into cubes
- ½ tsp of fresh paprika
- 3 cloves of minced garlic
- 4 oz (118 g) of white wine
- 2 tsp of fresh, minced rosemary
- 1 tbsp of olive oil
- 1 tbsp of mayonnaise
- ½ tsp of whole grain mustard
- 1 tsp of ground cinnamon
- 4 oz (123 g) of full-fat sour cream
- Salt and black pepper to taste

Instructions:

1. Put the chicken, white wine, and olive oil in a large bowl and stir to combine.
2. Add the cinnamon, smoked paprika, garlic, salt and pepper and work the ingredients into the chicken with your hands.
3. Cover with cling film and put the bowl in the fridge to marinate for 1 hour.
4. Set the air fryer to 375° F (190°C).
5. Transfer the chicken and the sauce into a baking dish.
6. Put the baking dish in the air fryer and cook for 20 minutes.
7. In a small bowl, add the sour cream, rosemary, mayonnaise, and mustard and stir to combine.
8. The chicken is cooked when the inside temperature is 165° F (74°C).
9. Once the chicken is cooked, remove from the air fryer and serve with the sauce.

Piri Piri Flavored Chicken Wings

Nutrition: Calories: 517, Protein: 4 g, Fats: 21 g, Carbs: 12 g, Fiber: 1 g

Total Time: 30 minutes

Servings: 2 (12 wings, 6 wings per person)

Ingredients For the Chicken

- 12 chicken wings
- 1 tsp of garlic paste
- ½ tsp of cumin powder
- 1 tsp of onion powder
- 1 oz (43 g) of melted butter

Ingredients For the Piri Piri Sauce

- ½ tsp of tarragon
- 1/3 tsp of sea salt
- 2 tbsp of fresh lemon juice
- 1 clove of chopped garlic
- 1 tbsp pimento seeds
- 2 oz (57 g) of piri piri peppers chopped and stemmed

Instructions:

1. In a large bowl, add the chicken wings, butter, garlic, cumin powder, and onion powder. Use your hands to work the ingredients into the chicken.
2. Set the air fryer to 330° F (166°C).
3. Cook the chicken for 20 minutes and turn halfway through.
4. Prepare the sauce by adding all the ingredients to a food processor and blend to combine.
5. Pour the sauce into two bowls.
6. Once the chicken is crispy and golden brown in color and the inside temperature is 165° F (74°C), serve with the piri piri sauce.

Roast Chicken Leg

Nutrition: Calories: 390, Protein: 12 g, Fats: 15 g, Carbs: 7 g, Fiber: 1 g

Total Time: 1 hour 30 minutes

Servings: 6

Ingredients:

- 6 skinless and boneless chicken legs
- 1 tsp of ground nutmeg
- 2 tbsp of olive oil
- ½ tsp of smoked cayenne pepper
- ½ tsp of fried oregano
- 3 cloves of minced garlic
- 2 chopped large tomatoes
- 2 sliced leeks
- Hoisin sauce

Instructions:

1. Put all the ingredients (except the leeks) into a large bowl and use your hands to combine everything.
2. Cover the bowl with cling film and put it in the fridge to marinate for one hour.
3. Set the air fryer to 375° F (191°C).
4. Arrange the leeks on the bottom of the air fryer basket.
5. Put the marinated chicken on top of the leeks and cook for 20 minutes.
6. Once the chicken has turned golden brown and crispy, and the inside temperature is 165° F (74°C), remove from the air fryer and serve with the hoisin sauce.

Chicken and Brussels Sprouts

Nutrition: Calories: 365, Protein: 14 g, Fats: 20 g, Carbs: 21 g, Fiber: 4 g

Total Time: 1 hour

Servings: 2

Ingredients:

- 2 chicken legs
- 8 oz (227 g) of Brussels sprouts
- 1 tsp of dried dill
- ½ tsp of black pepper
- ½ tsp of salt
- ½ tsp of paprika

Instructions:

1. Add the chicken legs, salt, pepper, and paprika to a medium sized bowl and use your hands to work the ingredients into the chicken.
2. In a separate bowl, season the Brussels sprouts with dill.
3. Set the air fryer to 370° F (188°C).
4. Put the chicken legs into the air fryer and cook for 10 minutes.
5. Set the air fryer to 380° F (193°C), add the Brussels sprouts and cook for 10 minutes.
6. Shake the basket halfway through.
7. Once the chicken is golden brown and crispy and the inside temperature is 165° F (74°C), remove it from the air fryer and serve.

Turnip With Chicken Legs

Nutrition: Calories: 207, Protein: 29 g, Fats: 7 g, Carbs: 3 g, Fiber: 1 g

Total Time: 1 hour

Servings: 3

Ingredients:

- 1 lb (454 g) of chicken legs
- 1 turnip sliced and trimmed
- 1 tsp of salt
- ½ tsp of ground black pepper
- 1 tsp of melted butter
- 1 tsp of paprika

Instructions:

1. Add the chicken legs, salt, pepper, and paprika to a medium sized bowl and use your hands to work the ingredients into the chicken.
2. In a separate medium sized bowl, drizzle the melted butter over the turnip and toss to combine.
3. Set the air fryer to 370° F (188°C).
4. Transfer the chicken to the air fryer and cook for 10 minutes.
5. Turn the temperature up to 380 F (193°C), add the turnips and cook for 15 minutes.
6. Flip the chicken and the turnips halfway through.
7. The chicken is cooked when the inside temperature is 165° F

(74 °C).

8. Once the chicken and the turnips are golden brown in color, remove from the air fryer and serve.

Chicken and Ham With Cheese

Nutrition: Calories: 480, Protein: 34 g, Fats: 36 g, Carbs: 4 g, Fiber: 0 g

Total Time: 40 minutes

Servings: 4

Ingredients:

- 8 oz (250 g) of cooked shredded chicken
- 4 oz (113 g) of chopped ham
- 4 oz (113 g) of sliced Swiss cheese
- 2 tbsp of white wine vinegar
- 1 tsp of Dijon mustard
- 4 oz (113 g) of softened cream cheese
- 2 oz (57 g) of softened unsalted butter
- Olive oil

Instructions:

1. In a large bowl, add the cream cheese, butter, white wine vinegar, and Dijon mustard and whisk together thoroughly.
2. Grease an 8-inch round baking pan with olive oil.
3. Place the chicken in the baking pan.
4. Put the ham on top of the chicken.
5. Spread the cream butter mixture over the ham.
6. Arrange the cheese slices over the top.
7. Put the baking pan into the air fryer and cook for 30 minutes.
8. The chicken is cooked when the inside temperature is 165° F (74°C).
9. The ham is cooked when the inside temperature is 145° F (63°C).
10. Once the cheese has browned, remove from the air fryer and serve.

You'll be spoilt for choice in this chapter with a wide selection of delightful juicy meaty recipes to engage your pallet.

Taco Rolls With Ground Beef

Nutrition: Calories: 380, Protein: 25 g, Fats: 26 g, Carbs: 5 g, Fiber: 2 g

Total Time: 30 minutes

Servings: 4

Ingredients:

- 1 large egg
- 2 oz (56 g) of cream cheese, full fat
- 1 oz (48 g) of blanched finely ground almond flour
- 12 oz (340 g) of shredded Mozzarella cheese
- 2 tbsp of chopped cilantro
- 2 oz (56 g), diced tomatoes and chilies, drained
- ¼ tsp of dried oregano
- ½ tsp of garlic powder
- 2 tsp of cumin
- 1 tbsp of chili powder
- 2 oz (79 g) of water
- ½ pound (227 g) of ground beef

Instructions:

1. Set the air fryer to 360° F (182° C).
2. In a medium sized saucepan over medium heat, brown the ground beef. The beef should be cooked within 10 minutes.
3. Drain the excess water from the beef and set it to one side.
4. In the same saucepan, add water, tomatoes with chilies, oregano, garlic powder, cumin, and chili powder and whisk to combine.
5. Leave the ingredients to simmer for 3 minutes, add the cilantro, stir to combine and remove the saucepan from the fire.
6. In a large microwavable bowl, combine the almond flour, cream cheese, Mozzarella cheese and egg and stir to combine.
7. Heat the mixture for 1 minute, remove from the microwave and stir to combine until a dough forms.
8. Sprinkle some flour on your work surface and roll out the dough until it's thick like a tortilla.
9. Divide the dough into 8 equal squares.
10. Spoon the beef mixture onto each of the eight squares and fold into a burrito.
11. Place a sheet of parchment paper into the air fryer basket.
12. Arrange the taco rolls in the air fryer and cook for 10 minutes.
13. Flip the tacos halfway through.
14. The beef is cooked when the inside temperature is 160° F (71° C).
15. Once the tacos are light brown in color, remove from the air fryer and serve with the sauce.

Seasoned Rack of Lamb

Nutrition: Calories: 645, Protein: 49 g, Fats: 48 g, Carbs: 1 g, Fiber: 0 g

Total Time: 25 minutes

Servings: 2

Ingredients:

- 14 oz (397 g) lamb rack
- ½ tsp of black pepper
- ½ tsp of salt
- 1 tsp of chopped fresh thyme
- 1 tsp of chopped fresh rosemary
- 1 tbsp of olive oil

Instructions:

1. Set the air fryer to 360° F (182° C).
2. In a large bowl, combine the rosemary, thyme, salt, pepper, and olive oil. Whisk together thoroughly.
3. Put the lamb rack into the bowl and season it.
4. Put the lamb rack into the air fryer and cook for 20 minutes.
5. The lamb is cooked when the inside temperature is 145° F (63° C), and it has turned golden brown in color.
6. Once cooked, remove the lamb rack from the air fryer, cover with foil and let it rest for 5 minutes before serving.

Lamb Kebabs With Coconut Curry Dipping Sauce

Nutrition: Calories: 262, Protein: 12 g, Fats: 23 g, Carbs: 2 g, Fiber: 1 g

Total Time: 25 minutes

Servings: 6

Ingredients For the Lamb Kebabs:

- 2 lb (907 g) of ground minced lamb
- 1 tsp of turmeric powder
- 1 tsp of ground cilantro
- 1 tsp of ground cumin
- 1 finely chopped spring onion
- 12 bamboo skewers soaked in water for 1 hour

Ingredients For the Coconut Curry Sauce:

- 2 tbsp of curry powder
- 9 oz (258 g) of coconut cream

Instructions

1. Set the air fryer to 400° F (204 ° C).
2. Add all the ingredients for the lamb kebabs to a large bowl and use your clean hands to combine and form into 12 kebabs.
3. Push the skewers through the kebabs.
4. Put the kebabs in the air fryer and cook for 15 minutes.
5. To make the dipping sauce, put the ingredients into a small bowl and whisk to combine.
6. The kebabs are cooked when they turn golden brown in color and the inside temperature is 145° F (63° C).
7. Once cooked, remove the kebabs from the air fryer and serve with the dipping sauce.

Beef Tenderloin Encrusted With Peppercorns

Nutrition: Calories: 289, Protein: 35 g, Fats: 17 g, Carbs: 2 g, Fiber: 1 g

Total Time: 35 minutes

Servings: 6

Ingredients:

- 2 lb (907 g) beef tenderloin, fat trimmed
- 3 tbsp of ground peppercorn blend
- 2 tsp of minced roasted garlic
- 2 tbsp of melted salted butter

Instructions:

1. Set the air fryer to 400° F (204° C).
2. In small bowl, combine the melted butter and roasted garlic.
3. Brush the butter mixture onto the beef tenderloin.
4. Roll the beef in the peppercorns and place them into a baking dish.
5. Put the baking dish in the air fryer and cook for 25 minutes.
6. Flip the beef tenderloin halfway through.
7. The beef tenderloin will be dark brown in color when cooked and the inside temperature is 160° F (71° C).
8. Once cooked, remove the beef tenderloin from the air fryer and leave it to rest for 10 minutes before slicing and serving.

Beef Stir-Fry With Broccoli

Nutrition: Calories: 342, Protein: 27 g, Fats: 19 g, Carbs: 10 g, Fiber: 3 g

Total Time: 35 minutes

Servings: 6

Ingredients:

- ½ tsp of sesame seeds
- 1/8 tsp of xanthan gum
- ¼ tsp of crushed red pepper
- 5 oz (142 g) of broccoli florets
- 1 tbsp of coconut oil
- ¼ tsp of finely minced garlic
- ¼ tsp of grated ginger
- 2 tbsp of coconut aminos
- ½ lb (227 g) of thinly sliced sirloin steak

Instructions:

1. Set the air fryer to 320° F (160° C).
2. Put the beef steak in a large bowl, add the coconut oil, garlic, ginger, and coconut aminos and use your clean hands to rub ingredients into the beef.
3. Remove the beef from the marinade and place it into a baking dish.
4. Put the baking dish in the air fryer and cook the beef for 20 minutes.
5. Flip the beef halfway through.
6. Add the red pepper and broccoli to the air fryer for the last 10 minutes of cooking.
7. Transfer the marinade into a saucepan and simmer on low heat.
8. Add the xanthan gum to thicken and stir to combine.
9. The beef will be dark brown in color when it's cooked, the inside temperature will be 160° F (71° C), and the vegetables

will be tender.

10. Once cooked, remove the beef and vegetables from the air fryer, sprinkle with sesame seeds and serve.

Baby Spareribs

Nutrition: Calories: 466, Protein: 49 g, Fats: 28 g, Carbs: 1 g, Fiber: 0 g

Total Time: 30 minutes

Servings: 4

Ingredients:

- 4.2 oz (120 g) of sugar-free, low-carb barbeque sauce
- ¼ tsp of ground cayenne pepper
- ½ tsp of garlic powder
- ½ tsp of onion powder
- 1 tsp of paprika
- 2 tsp of chili powder
- 2 lb (907 g) of baby back ribs

Instructions:

1. Set the air fryer to 400° F (204° C).
2. Put the ribs into a baking dish and add all the ingredients except the barbeque sauce.
3. With clean hands, rub the ingredients into the ribs.
4. Put the baking dish into the air fryer and cook for 25 minutes.
5. The ribs will be dark brown in color when cooked and the inside temperature will be 190° F (88° C).
6. Once cooked, remove the ribs from the air fryer, coat in the barbeque sauce and serve.

Lamb Chops With Mojito Marinade

Nutrition: Calories: 692, Protein: 48 g, Fats: 53 g, Carbs: 4 g, Fiber: 1 g

Total Time: 15 minutes

Servings: 2

Ingredients For the Lamb Chops:

- 4 lamb chops
- ½ tsp of black pepper
- 2 tsp of sea salt

Ingredients For the Marinade

- 4 cloves of chopped garlic
- .2 oz (6 g) of chopped fresh mint leaves
- .2 oz (6 g) of avocado oil
- 4 oz (115 g) of lime juice
- 2 tsp of grated lime zest

Ingredients For Garnish

- 1 lime sliced into rounds
- Sprigs of fresh mint

Instructions:

1. Put all the ingredients for the marinade into a food processor and pulse until smooth but chunky.
2. Place the lamb chops in a shallow dish.
3. Pour half of the marinade, salt , black pepper over the lamb chops and put the rest to one side.
4. Leave the lamb chops in the fridge overnight.

5. Set the air fryer to 390° F (200° C).

6. Take the lamb chops out of the fridge, place them into the air fryer and cook for 5 minutes.

7. The lamb chops are cooked when the inside temperature reaches 145° F (63° C), and they are golden brown in color.

8. Once the lamb chops are cooked, remove them from the air fryer and let them rest for ten minutes.

9. Pour the remaining marinade over the lamb chops, garnish with lime and mint and serve.

Pork Meatballs

Nutrition: Calories: 164, Protein: 15 g, Fats: 10 g, Carbs: 1 g, Fiber: 0 g

Total Time: 25 minutes

Servings: 18 meatballs (6 per person)

Ingredients:

- 1 medium scallion, sliced and trimmed
- ¼ tsp of crushed red pepper flakes
- ½ tsp of ground ginger
- ½ tsp of salt
- ½ tsp of garlic powder
- 1 large egg
- 1 lb (454 g) of ground pork

Instructions:

1. Set the air fryer at 400° F (204° C).

2. Put all the ingredients into a large bowl, use your clean hands to combine everything together.

3. Form the ingredients into meatballs.

4. Arrange the meatballs into a baking dish.

5. Put the baking dish into the air Fryer and cook for 12 minutes.

6. Shake the basket halfway through.

7. The meatballs are cooked when they turn golden brown in color and the inside temperature is 145° F (63° C).

8. Once cooked, remove the meatballs from the air fryer and serve.

Sweet & Sour Pork

Nutrition: Calories: 304, Protein: 31 g, Fats: 10 g, Carbs: 22 g, Fiber: 0 g

Total Time: 35 minutes

Servings: 4

Ingredients For the Pork:

- 1 lb (680 g) of pork cutlets sliced into 1-inch pieces
- 3 tbsp of cornstarch
- Avocado oil cooking spray

Ingredients For the Sauce:

- 2 tbsp of soy sauce
- 4 tbsp of ketchup
- 2 oz (58 g) of rice vinegar
- 1 oz (50 g) of white sugar

Instructions:

1. Set the air fryer to 350° F (177° C).

2. Combine the pork and the cornstarch in a large bowl and toss to coat.

3. Spray the pork with cooking spray.

4. Put the pork into a baking dish and put it into the air fryer and cook for 10 minutes.

5. Shake the basket half way through.

6. In a small saucepan, add the sugar, soy sauce, ketchup, and vinegar to, whisk to combine and heat over a medium temperature stirring constantly until the sugar melts.

7. Turn the heat down to low and let it simmer until the pork is ready.

8. The pork is ready when it has an inside temperature of 160° F (71° C), and its golden brown in color.

9. Once the pork is cooked, remove it from the air fryer and serve with the sweet & sour sauce.

Shredded Beef Mexican Style

Nutrition: Calories: 217, Protein: 37 g, Fats: 6 g, Carbs: 0 g, Fiber: 0 g

Total Time: 40 minutes

Servings: 6

Ingredients:

- 3 oz (100 g) of sugar-free chipotle sauce
- ½ tsp of ground black pepper
- 1 tsp of salt
- 2 lb (907 g) of beef chuck roast sliced into 2-inch cubes

Instructions:

1. Set the air fryer to 400° F (204° C).

2. Put the beef into a baking dish and season with salt and pepper.

3. Put the baking dish in the air fryer and cook for 30 minutes.

4. The beef is cooked when it turns dark brown in color and it has an inside temperature of 160° F (71° C).

5. Remove the baking dish from the air fryer and shred with two forks.

6. Add the chipotle sauce and toss to combine.

Parmesan Flavored Pork Chops

Nutrition: Calories: 298, Protein: 29 g, Fats: 17 g, Carbs: 2 g, Fiber: 0 g

Total Time: 20 minutes

Servings: 4

Ingredients:

- ¼ tsp of ground black pepper
- ½ tsp of salt
- 4 oz (113 g) of boneless pork chops
- 1 oz (45 g) of Parmesan cheese, grated
- 1 large egg

Instructions:

1. Set the air fryer to 400° F (204° C).

2. Whisk the egg in a medium sized bowl.

3. Put the Parmesan cheese in a medium sized bowl.

4. Put the pork chops in a baking dish and season with salt and pepper.

5. Dip the pork chops into the egg and then the Parmesan.

6. Put the pork chops back into the baking dish and then into the air fryer.

7. Cook the pork chops for 12 minutes.

8. Turn the pork chops halfway through.

9. The pork chops will be dark brown in color when cooked with an inside temperature of 145° F (63° C).

10. Once cooked, remove the pork chops from the air fryer and serve.

Seasoned Pork Chops

Nutrition: Calories: 454, Protein: 33 g, Fats: 31 g, Carbs: 11 g, Fiber: 2 g

Total Time: 1 hour 30 minutes

Servings: 4

Ingredients:

- 1 pound (454 g) of pork chops
- Salt and pepper to taste
- ¼ tsp of cayenne pepper
- ½ tsp of onion powder
- 1 tsp of smoked paprika
- 1 tbsp of avocado oil

Instructions:

1. Set the air fryer to 400° F (204° C).

2. In a large bowl, combine the salt, pepper, cayenne pepper, onion powder, and smoked paprika.

3. Brush the pork chops with avocado oil.

4. Dip the pork chops in the seasoning mix.

5. Arrange the pork chops in the air fryer and cook for 12 minutes.

6. Flip the pork chops halfway through.

7. The pork chops will be golden brown in color and have an inside temperature of 145° F (63° C) when cooked.

8. Once cooked, remove the pork chops from the air fryer and serve.

Simple Lamb Kofta

Nutrition: Calories: 437, Protein: 38 g, Fats: 27 g, Carbs: 2 g, Fiber: 1 g

Total Time: 30 minutes

Servings: 6

Ingredients:

- 2 lb (907 g) of ground lamb
- ½ tsp of black pepper
- ½ tsp of ground cinnamon
- ¾ tsp of salt
- 1 tsp of paprika
- 1 tbsp of ground cumin
- 1 tbsp of ground coriander
- 2 tbsp of chopped fresh cilantro
- 2 cloves of finely chopped garlic
- 12 bamboo skewers soaked in water for 1 hour

Instructions:

1. Set the air fryer to 400° F (204° C).

2. Add all the ingredients to a large bowl and use your clean hands to combine.

3. Roll the mixture into 12 oval shaped logs about 4 inches long and 1 inch wide.

4. Thread 1 log through each skewer.

5. Put the lamb into the air fryer and cook for 10 minutes.

6. The lamb is cooked when it reaches an inside temperature of 135° F (57° C), and they turn golden brown in color.

7. Once cooked, remove the lamb from the air fryer and leave it to rest for 5 minutes before serving.

Peppers Stuffed With Sausage

Nutrition: Calories: 186, Protein: 11 g, Fats: 12 g, Carbs: 8 g, Fiber: 2 g

Total Time: 45 minutes

Servings: 6

Ingredients:

- 3 oz (85 g) of shredded provolone cheese
- 3 bell peppers, seeded and cut in halves
- 8 oz (227 g) of keto-friendly Mariana sauce
- Salt and pepper
- 1 tsp of Italian seasoning
- ½ oz (14 g) of diced onion
- .8 oz (25 g) of sliced mushrooms
- 8 oz (227 g) of Italian sausage casings removed
- Avocado oil spray

Instructions:

1. Set the air fryer to 350° F (177 ° C).

2. Spray a large frying pan with avocado oil.

3. Cook the sausage over medium temperature for 5 minutes at the same time as breaking it up.

4. Season the sausage with salt and pepper.

5. Add the mushrooms, onions, and Italian seasoning and stir to combine.

6. Add the marinara sauce and stir to combine.

7. Turn the temperature down to low and leave the ingredients to cook for 5 minutes.

8. Spoon the sausage mixture into the bell pepper halves.

9. Put the stuffed bell peppers into the air fryer and cook for 15 minutes.

10. After 5 minutes, sprinkle the cheese over the top of the bell peppers.

11. The bell peppers are cooked once they turn soft and the cheese has melted.

12. The sausage is cooked when it has an internal temperature of 155 -165° F (74° C).

13. Once the bell peppers are cooked, remove them from the air fryer and serve.

Rosemary Flavored Roast Beef

Nutrition: Calories: 213, Protein: 25 g, Fats: 10 g, Carbs: 2 g, Fiber: 1 g

Total Time: 13 hours 35 minutes

Servings: 6

Ingredients:

- 2 oz (56 g) of avocado oil
- 2 tbsp of fresh, finely chopped rosemary
- 2 tsp of finely chopped garlic
- 1 lb (454 g) of top round beef roast, tied with kitchen string
- Salt and pepper to taste

Instructions:

1. Place the roast beef in a large bowl and season with salt and pepper.

2. In a small bowl, combine the avocado oil, rosemary, and garlic and whisk together.

3. Rub the rosemary mixture over the beef.

4. Loosely cover the roast beef with foil and put it in the fridge for 12 hours.

5. Take the roast beef out of the fridge and let it sit in room temperature for 1 hour.

6. Set the air fryer to 325° F (163 ° C).

7. Put the roast beef into the air fryer and cook it for 15 minutes.

8. Flip the roast beef and cook it for another 15 minutes.

9. The roast beef is ready when it turns golden brown in color and it has an inside temperature of 120° F (49° C).

10. Once the roast beef is cooked, remove it from the air fryer and let it rest for 15 minutes before serving.

Cheese & Herb Flavored Lamb Chops

Nutrition: Calories: 790, Protein: 57 g, Fats: 60 g, Carbs: 2 g, Fiber: 1 g

Total Time: 15 minutes

Servings: 2

Ingredients:

- 4 lamb chops
- ½ tsp of ground black pepper
- 1 tsp of chopped fresh thyme leaves
- 1 tbsp of fresh chopped rosemary leaves
- 1 tbsp of fresh chopped oregano leaves
- .8 oz (23 g) of powdered Parmesan cheese
- .3 oz (8 g) of pork dust
- 2 cloves of minced garlic
- 1 large egg
- Avocado oil spray

Ingredients For the Garnish

- 1 lemon sliced into rounds
- Lavender flowers
- Sprigs of fresh thyme
- Sprigs of fresh rosemary
- Sprigs of fresh oregano

Instructions:

1. Spray the air fryer basket with avocado oil.

2. Set the air fryer to 400° F (204° C).

3. In a small shallow bowl, whisk the egg and garlic.

4. In a separate small shallow bowl, combine the Parmesan cheese, pork dust, oregano, rosemary, thyme, and black pepper.

5. One by one, dip the lamb chops into the egg mixture and then into the Parmesan mixture. Use your clean hands to press the mixture into the lamb chops.

6. Put the lamb chops into the air fryer and cook for 5 minutes.

7. The lamb chops are cooked when the inside temperature reaches 145° F (63° C), and the outside is crispy and golden brown in color.

8. Once cooked, remove the lamb chops from the air fryer and leave them to rest for 10 minutes.

9. Top the lamb chops with the garnish and serve.

Chapter 7: Fish and Seafood Main Dishes

The rich, delicate flavors of seafood and fish make them the perfect choice for meatless Mondays or pescatarians.

Old Bay Tuna Patties

Nutrition: Calories: 100, Protein: 21 g, Fats: 2 g, Carbs: 1 g, Fiber: 0 g

Total Time: 20 minutes

Servings: 4

Ingredients:

- ½ tsp of old bay seasoning, salt
- 2 tbsp of white onion, chopped
- 1 large egg
- 4 pouches of tuna, drained

Instructions:

1. Set the air fryer to 400° F (204° C).
2. Transfer all the ingredients into a large bowl and stir to combine.
3. Shape the mixture into 4 patties.
4. Put the patties into the air fryer and cook for 10 minutes.
5. The patties will be golden brown in color and they will have an inside temperature of 125° F (52° C) when cooked.
6. Once cooked, remove the patties from the air fryer and serve.

Cajun Salmon Patties

Nutrition: Calories: 263, Protein: 20 g, Fats: 18 g, Carbs: 2 g, Fiber: 3 g

Total Time: 15 minutes

Servings: 4

Ingredients:

- 1 medium avocado, skin removed, deseeded, and sliced
- ½ tsp of Cajun seasoning, salt
- 1 oz (28 g) of blanched finely ground almond flour
- 3 tbsp of mayonnaise
- 1 pouch of pink salmon (12 oz or 340 g)

Instructions:

1. Set the air fryer to 400° F (204° C).
2. In a large bowl, combine all the ingredients and form four patties.
3. Put the patties into the air fryer and cook for 8 minutes.
4. Turn the patties over halfway through.
5. The patties are cooked once they turn golden brown in color and have an inside temperature of 145° F (63° C).
6. Once cooked, remove the patties from the air fryer and serve.

Spicy & Sweet Salmon

Nutrition: Calories: 326, Protein: 23 g, Fats: 25 g, Carbs: 1 g, Fiber: 0 g

Total Time: 25 minutes

Servings: 4

Ingredients:

- 16 oz (454 g) of salmon fillets
- 1 tsp of adobo sauce

- 1 diced chipotle chili in adobo sauce
- 2 tsp of Dijon mustard
- 2 tbsp of Swerve
- 4 oz (115 g) of sugar-free mayonnaise
- Salt and pepper for seasoning

Instructions:

1. Set the air fryer to 400° F (204° C).
2. Add the adobo sauce, chipotle pepper, Dijon mustard, sugar-free mayonnaise, salt, pepper and Swerve to a food processor and blend until smooth.
3. Arrange the salmon in a baking pan and pour half the blended sauce over the top.
4. Leave the other half of the sauce for dipping.
5. Put the baking pan in the air fryer and cook for 7 minutes.
6. The salmon will have an inside temperature of 145° F (63° C) when cooked.
7. Once cooked, remove the salmon from the air fryer.
8. Warm the sauce in the microwave and serve.

Stuffed Florentine Flounder

Nutrition: Calories: 311, Protein: 31 g, Fats: 18 g, Carbs: 9 g, Fiber: 1 g

Total Time: 35 minutes

Servings: 4

Ingredients:

- ½ a lemon cut into 4 wedges
- A dash of paprika
- 4 flounder fillets
- 2 tbsp of unsalted butter
- Salt and pepper for seasoning
- 2 cloves of chopped garlic
- 1 bag of spinach (170 g or 6 oz) roughly chopped
- 3 oz (100 g) of chopped tomatoes
- 2 tbsp of olive oil
- 1 oz (34 g) of pine nuts

Instructions:

1. Set the air fryer to 400° F (204° C)
2. Put the pine nuts into a baking dish.
3. Put the baking dish into the air fryer and cook the pine nuts for 4 minutes.
4. Once the pine nuts are slightly brown, remove them from the air fryer and leave them to one side.
5. Add the spinach, garlic, tomatoes, paprika and olive oil to a baking dish and toss to combine.
6. Put the baking dish in the air fryer and cook for 5 minutes.
7. Once the spinach is wilted and the tomatoes are soft, remove the baking dish from the air fryer.
8. Add the pine nuts and the roasted vegetables to a large bowl and toss to combine.
9. Turn the air fryer down to 350° F (177° C).

10. Grease a baking dish with 2 tablespoon of butter.
11. Lay the flounder in the baking dish and top with the vegetable mixture with salt and pepper .
12. Roll each piece of flounder and secure with a toothpick.
13. Put the baking dish in the air fryer and cook for 15 minutes.
14. The flounder will have an inside temperature of 145° F (62° C) when cooked.
15. Once cooked, remove the baking tray from the air fryer, and serve with lemon wedges.

Catfish Encrusted With Pecans

Nutrition: Calories: 162, Protein: 17 g, Fats: 11 g, Carbs: 0 g, Fiber: 1 g

Total Time: 20 minutes

Servings: 4

Ingredients:

- 4 catfish fillets
- ¼ tsp of ground black pepper
- 1 tsp of fine sea salt
- .8 oz (24 g) of pecan meal
- Avocado oil spray
- For garnish: Pecan halves,
- For garnish: Fresh oregano

Instructions:

1. Set the air fryer to 350° F (177° C).
2. In a large bowl, add the pecan meal, salt and pepper and toss to combine.
3. Dip the catfish fillets into the pecan meal mixture and press in with your hands.
4. Spray the catfish with avocado oil.
5. Transfer the coated catfish into the air fryer and cook for 12 minutes.
6. Flip the fish halfway through.
7. The catfish will have an inside temperature of 145° F (63° C) when cooked.
8. Once the catfish is cooked, remove them from the air fryer, top with pecan halves and oregano and serve.

Salmon Kebabs

Nutrition: Calories: 183, Protein: 17 g, Fats: 9 g, Carbs: 6 g, Fiber: 1 g

Total Time: 20 minutes

Servings: 4

Ingredients:

- ¼ tsp of ground black pepper
- ½ tsp of salt
- 1 tbsp of olive oil
- ½ a medium zucchini, cut into ½ inch slices and trimmed
- ½ a medium yellow pepper, sliced into 1-inch pieces and seeds removed
- ¼ medium red onion sliced into 1-inch pieces
- 6 oz (170 g) of skinless, boneless salmon, sliced into 1-inch cubes
- 4 wooden skewers, 6-inches

Instructions:

1. Set the air fryer to 400° F (204° C).
2. Thread a piece of salmon, onion, bell pepper and zucchini through a skewer.
3. Repeat for the remaining skewers.
4. Season the kebabs with salt and pepper.
5. Coat kebabs with olive oil.
6. Put the kebabs into the air fryer and cook for 8 minutes.
7. Turn the kebabs over halfway through.
8. The vegetables will be tender and the salmon flaky when cooked.
9. The salmon is cooked when it reaches an inside temperature of 145° F (63° C).
10. Once cooked, remove the kebabs from the air fryer and served.

Avocado Boats Stuffed With Crab

Nutrition: Calories: 209, Protein: 12 g, Fats: 15 g, Carbs: 1 g, Fiber: 2 g

Total Time: 15 minutes

Servings: 4

Ingredients:

- 2 tbsp mayonnaise
- 2 tbsp diced yellow onion
- ¼ tsp of Old Bay seasoning
- 8 oz (227 g) of cooked crab meat
- 2 medium avocados, cut in halves and seeds removed

Instructions:

1. Set the air fryer to 350° F (177° C).
2. Spoon the avocado flesh out of the skin and put the flesh to one side.
3. In a medium sized bowl combine the crab meat, Old Bay seasoning, onion, and mayonnaise.
4. Full the avocado halves with the mixture and put them into the air fryer.
5. Cook the stuffed avocados for 7 minutes.
6. When the stuffed avocados are cooked, the mixture on top will be browned and bubbly.
7. The crab is cooked when it reaches an inside temperature of 145° F (63° C).
8. Once cooked, remove the stuffed avocados from the air fryer and serve.

Shrimp Flavored With Lime and Chili

Nutrition: Calories: 98, Protein: 13 g, Fats: 4 g, Carbs: 1 g, Fiber: 1 g

Total Time: 10 minutes

Servings: 4

Ingredients:

- The juice of half a small lime
- The zest of half a small lime
- ¼ tsp of ground black pepper
- ¼ tsp of salt
- ¼ tsp of garlic powder

- 2 tsp of chili powder
- 1 tbsp of salted melted butter
- 1 pound (453 g) of shrimp, deveined and peeled

Instructions:

1. Set the air fryer to 300° F (149° C).

2. In a medium sized bowl, combine the shrimp, butter, lime zest, salt, pepper, garlic powder, and chili powder, and toss to coat.

3. Transfer the shrimp into a baking dish.

4. Put the baking dish into the air fryer and cook for 5 minutes.

5. The shrimp will be dark pink in color once cooked and it has an inside temperature of 145° F (63° C).

6. Remove the shrimp from the air fryer, drizzle with lime juice and serve.

Seasoned Tuna Steaks

Nutrition: Calories: 385, Protein: 0 g, Fats: 14 g, Carbs: 0 g, Fiber: 0 g

Total Time: 20 minutes

Servings: 2

Ingredients:

- 3 tbsp of Everything bagel seasoning, salt
- 2 tbsp of olive oil
- 2 oz (170 g) tuna steaks

Instructions:

1. Set the air fryer to 400° F (204° C).

2. Arrange the tuna steaks on a baking tray and brush with olive oil and salt.

3. Sprinkle the seasoning over the tuna steaks.

4. Put the tuna steaks into the air fryer and cook for 14 minutes.

5. Flip the tuna steaks halfway through.

6. The tuna steaks will be cooked once they are golden brown in color and they have an inside temperature of 145° F (63° C).

7. Once cooked, remove the tuna steaks from the air fryer and serve.

Garlic Buttered Crab Legs

Nutrition: Calories: 123, Protein: 6 g, Fats: 6 g, Carbs: 0 g, Fiber: 0 g

Total Time: 20 minutes

Servings: 4

Ingredients:

- The juice of ½ a lemon
- ¼ tsp of garlic powder
- 3 lb (1360 g) of crab legs
- 2 oz (60 g) of melted salted butter

Instructions:

1. Put the crab legs into a large bowl and coat them with 2 tablespoons of butter.

2. Transfer the crab legs into a baking dish.

3. Put the baking dish into the air fryer.

4. Set the air fryer to 300° F (149° C).

5. Cook the crab legs for 15 minutes.

6. Shake the air fryer basket halfway through.

7. In a small bowl, combine the lemon juice, remaining butter, and garlic powder and whisk together thoroughly.

8. The crab is cooked when it has an inside temperature of 145° F (63° C).

9. Once the crab legs are cooked, remove them from the air fryer and serve with the butter dip.

Crunchy Fish Sticks

Nutrition: Calories: 205, Protein: 24 g, Fats: 10 g, Carbs: 2 g, Fiber: 1 g

Total Time: 20 minutes

Servings: 4

Ingredients:

- 1 lb (454 g) of cod fillets sliced into ¾ inch strips
- 1 large egg
- 1 tbsp of coconut oil
- ½ tsp of Old Bay seasoning, salt
- .8 oz (24 g) of blanched finely ground almond flour
- 1 oz (28 g) of finely ground pork rinds

Instructions:

1. In a large bowl, add the almond flour, Old Bay seasoning, salt, pork rinds, and coconut oil and stir to combine.

2. Whisk the egg in a medium sized bowl.

3. Dip the cod fillets into the egg and then into the flour mixture.

4. Arrange the cod fillets into a baking dish.

5. Set the air fryer to 300° F (148° C).

6. Put the baking dish into the air fryer and cook for 10 minutes.

7. The cod fillets are cooked once they turn golden brown in color and they have an inside temperature of 145° F (63° C).

8. Once cooked, remove the cod fillets from the air fryer and serve.

Cajun Flavored Haddock

Nutrition: Calories: 253, Protein: 21 g, Fats: 16 g, Carbs: 2 g, Fiber: 1 g

Total Time: 15 minutes

Servings: 2

Ingredients:

- ¼ tsp of ground black pepper, salt
- 1 tsp of paprika
- ½ tsp of garlic powder
- 1/8 tsp of ground cayenne pepper
- 2 tbsp of melted unsalted butter
- 4 oz (113 g) skinless haddock fillets

Instructions:

1. Set the air fryer to 300° F (149° C).

2. Brush the fillets with melted butter.

3. Add the cayenne pepper, garlic powder, paprika, salt and black pepper to a small bowl and toss to combine.

4. Season the haddock with the mixture and place it into a baking dish.

5. Put the baking dish into the air fryer and cook for 7 minutes.

6. The haddock will be golden brown in color once cooked with an inside temperature of 145° F (63° C).

7. Remove the haddock from the air fryer and serve.

Cod Sticks With Tartar Sauce

Nutrition: Calories: 600, Protein: 5 g, Fats: 42 g, Carbs: 14 g, Fiber: 2 g

Total Time: 30 minutes

Servings: 4

Ingredients For the Cod Sticks:

- 1 lb (454 g) of cod fillets sliced into 1-inch strips
- .8 oz (23 g) of grated Parmesan cheese
- 2 oz (72 g) of almond flour
- 2 eggs
- ½ tsp of ground black pepper
- 1 tsp of salt
- Avocado oil

Ingredients For the Tartar Sauce

- 1 tbsp of Dill pickle liquid
- ½ tsp of dried dill
- 2 tbsp of capers chopped and drained
- 3 tbsp of chopped Dill pickle
- 4 oz (115 g) of mayonnaise
- 4 oz (115 g) of sour cream

Instructions:

1. Set the air fryer to 400° F (204° C).
2. Season the cod with salt and pepper and put it to one side.
3. Lightly whisk the eggs in a shallow bowl.
4. In another shallow bowl, combine the Parmesan cheese and almond flour, stir together thoroughly.
5. One at a time, dip the cod sticks into the egg and then into the Parmesan mix. Using clean hands, press the mixture into the cod sticks.
6. Spray the cod sticks with avocado oil and place them into the air fryer.
7. Cook the cod sticks for 15 minutes.
8. Flip the cod sticks halfway through.
9. Make the tartar sauce by combining all the ingredients into a small bowl and whisk to combine.
10. The cod sticks are cooked when they become crispy and golden brown in color, with an inside temperature of 145° F (63° C).
11. Once cooked, remove the cod sticks from the air fryer and serve with the tartar sauce.

Parmesan Flavored Lobster Tails

Nutrition: Calories: 184, Protein: 23 g, Fats: 9 g, Carbs: 1 g, Fiber: 0 g

Total Time: 15 minutes

Servings: 4

Ingredients:

- 4 oz (114 g) of lobster tails
- ½ oz (14 g) of finely crushed plain pork rinds
- .8 oz (23 g) of grated Parmesan cheese
- ¼ tsp of ground black pepper
- ¼ tsp of salt
- 1 tsp of Cajun seasoning
- 2 tbsp of melted salted butter

Instructions:

1. Set the air fryer to 400° F (204° C).
2. Use a pair of scissors to gently cut open the lobster tails and carefully pull the meat away from the shells. Rest the meat on top of the shells.
3. Brush the butter over the lobster meat.
4. Season the lobster meat with half of the Cajun seasoning.
5. In a small bowl, mix the pork rinds, Parmesan cheese, Cajun seasoning, and salt and stir to combine.
6. Roll the lobster meat into the mixture, and gently press it into the meat with clean hands.
7. Put the lobster meat into the air fryer and cook for 7 minutes.
8. The lobster tails are cooked when they turn crispy and golden brown in color and it has an inside temperature of 145° F (63° C).
9. Once cooked, remove the lobster tails from the air fryer and serve.

Cheesy Tuna Stuffed in Tomatoes

Nutrition: Calories: 219, Protein: 18 g, Fats: 15 g, Carbs: 4 g, Fiber: 1 g

Total Time: 15 minutes

Servings: 2

Ingredients:

- .8 oz (23 g) shredded Cheddar cheese
- 2 tsp of coconut oil
- ¼ tsp of ground black pepper
- ¼ tsp of salt
- 2 tbsp of mayonnaise
- 1 medium celery stalk, chopped and trimmed
- 2 pouches of tuna, drained
- 2 medium beefsteak tomatoes, tops, membranes, and seeds removed

Instructions:

1. Set the air fryer to 350° F (177° C).
2. In a large bowl, add the tuna, mayonnaise, celery, salt, pepper, and coconut oil and stir to combine.
3. Spoon the mixture into each tomato.
4. Top with Cheddar cheese.
5. Put the tomatoes in the air fryer and cook for 5 minutes.
6. The tomatoes are ready when the cheese is melted, and bubbling.
7. The tuna is cooked when it has an inside temperature of 145° F (63° C).
8. Once the tomatoes are cooked, remove them from the air fryer and serve.

Chapter 8: Vegetables and Sides

Pair these vegetables and sides with many of the other recipes including poultry, fish, beef, lamb, or pork.

Crunchy Green Beans

Nutrition: Calories: 37, Protein: 1 g, Fats: 2 g, Carbs: 2 g, Fiber: 2 g

Total Time: 15 minutes

Servings: 4

Ingredients:

- 8 oz (227g) of fresh green beans, trimmed ends
- 2 tsp of olive oil
- ¼ tsp of ground black pepper
- ¼ tsp of salt

Instructions:

1. Set the air fryer to 350° F (177° C).
2. Add all the ingredients to a large bowl and toss to combine.
3. Transfer the green beans into a baking dish.
4. Put the baking dish in the air fryer and cook for 8 minutes.
5. Shake the basket halfway through.
6. When cooked, the green beans will have a deep golden-brown color.
7. Once cooked, remove the green beans from the air fryer and serve.

Creamy Asparagus

Nutrition: Calories: 221, Protein: 7 g, Fats: 18 g, Carbs: 5 g, Fiber: 2 g

Total Time: 30 minutes

Servings: 4

Ingredients:

- 1 lb (454 g) of asparagus, sliced into 1-inch pieces with ends trimmed
- 2 oz (57 g) of softened cream cheese
- 1 oz (45 g) of grated Parmesan cheese
- 4.2 oz (120 g) of heavy whipping cream
- ¼ tsp of ground black pepper
- ¼ tsp of salt

Instructions:

1. Set the air fryer to 350° F (177° C).
2. Add the cream cheese, Parmesan, heavy whipping cream, salt, and pepper to a medium sized bowl and whisk to combine.
3. Put the asparagus into a baking dish and pour the cream mixture over the top.
4. Put the baking dish in the air fryer and cook for 18 minutes.
5. The asparagus are cooked once they become slightly soft.
6. Once cooked, remove the asparagus from the air fryer and serve.

Fried Asparagus

Nutrition: Calories: 73, Protein: 2 g, Fats: 6 g, Carbs: 2 g, Fiber: 2 g

Total Time: 20 minutes

Servings: 4

Ingredients:

- 1 lb (454 g) of asparagus spears, trimmed ends
- 1 tbsp of salted melted butter
- ¼ tsp of ground black pepper
- ¼ tsp of salt
- 1 tbsp of olive oil

Instructions:

1. Set the air fryer to 375° F (190° C).
2. Put the asparagus into a large bowl and toss with, melted butter, olive oil and salt and pepper.
3. Transfer the asparagus to a baking tray.
4. Put the baking tray into the air fryer and cook for 12 minutes.
5. The asparagus are cooked when they turn golden brown in color.
6. Once the asparagus are cooked, remove them from the air fryer and serve.

Balsamic Vinegar Flavored Brussels Sprouts

Nutrition: Calories: 112, Protein: 3 g, Fats: 9 g, Carbs: 5 g, Fiber: 2 g

Total Time: 20 minutes

Servings: 4

Ingredients:

- 2 tbsp of balsamic vinegar
- ¼ tsp of ground black pepper
- ¼ tsp of salt
- 2 tbsp of olive oil
- 6.2 oz (176 g) fresh Brussels sprouts, trimmed and cut in halves

Instructions:

1. Set the air fryer to 375° F (190° C).
2. In a large bowl, combine the Brussels sprouts, olive oil, balsamic vinegar, salt and pepper, and toss together.
3. Transfer the Brussels sprouts into a baking dish.
4. Put the baking dish into the air fryer and cook for 12 minutes.
5. The Brussels sprouts are cooked once they become caramelized and tender.

Zucchini Fritters

Nutrition: Calories: 190, Protein: 6 g, Fats: 16 g, Carbs: 8 g, Fiber: 2 g

Total Time: 20 minutes

Servings: 4

Ingredients:

- ½ a lemon, cut into wedges

- 1 tbsp of olive oil
- ¼ tsp of ground black pepper
- 1/4 tsp of turmeric
- ¼ tsp of dried thyme
- 1 large egg
- .8 oz (23 g) Parmesan cheese, grated
- .8 oz (23 g) of almond flour
- 1 tsp of salt
- 2 grated zucchinis

Instructions:

1. Set the air fryer to 300° F (149° C).
2. Lay a sheet of parchment paper in the air fryer basket.
3. Sprinkle salt over the zucchini and let it sit for 10 minutes to soak up the excess water.
4. Squeeze the remaining water out of the zucchini and put them to one side.
5. In a large bowl, combine the almond flour, egg, Parmesan, black pepper, turmeric, and thyme. Stir to combine to make a dough.
6. Knead the dough out on a work surface and cut into two even parts.
7. Roll the zucchini in the dough and brush with olive oil.
8. Place the zucchini fritters in the air fryer and cook for 10 minutes.
9. Flip the zucchini fritters halfway through.
10. The zucchini fritters are cooked when they turn golden brown in color.
11. Once cooked, remove the zucchini fritters from the air fryer and serve with lemon wedges.

Brussels Sprouts With Gorgonzola & Pecans

Nutrition: Calories: 250, Protein: 9 g, Fats: 19 g, Carbs: 9 g, Fiber: 8 g

Total Time: 35 minutes

Servings: 4

Ingredients:

- 1 oz (30 g) of Gorgonzola cheese
- Salt and pepper for seasoning
- 2 tbsp of olive oil
- 1 lb (680 g) of fresh Brussels sprouts, trimmed and quartered
- 2.11 oz (60 g) of pecans

Instructions:

1. Set the air fryer to 350° F (177° C).
2. Add the pecans to the air fryer and cook for three minutes.
3. The pecans are cooked once they've turned golden brown in color.
4. Remove the pecans from the air fryer and put them to one side.
5. Turn up the air fryer to 400° F (204° C).
6. Add the Brussels sprouts to a large bowl and toss with olive oil and salt and pepper.
7. Transfer the Brussels sprouts into a baking dish.
8. Put the baking dish in the air fryer and cook for 20 minutes,
9. The Brussels sprouts are cooked once they become tender and turn brown around the edges.

10. Once cooked, remove the Brussels sprouts from the air fryer, sprinkle with pine nuts and cheese and serve.

Roasted Salsa

Nutrition: Calories: 28, Protein: 1 g, Fats: 2 g, Carbs: 2 g, Fiber: 1 g

Total Time: 45 minutes

Servings: 2 cups

Ingredients:

- 2 oz (57 g) of fresh lime juice
- 1 tbsp of coconut oil
- ½ tsp of salt
- 2 cloves of diced garlic
- ½ a medium jalapeno, diced and seeds removed
- ½ a diced medium white onion
- 2 large San Marzano tomatoes, sliced into large chunks and cored

Instructions:

1. Set the air fryer to 300° F (149 ° C).
2. In a large baking dish, add the tomatoes, coconut oil, salt, garlic, jalapeno, and onion and toss to combine.
3. Put the baking dish into the air fryer and cook for 30 minutes.
4. The vegetables are cooked once they become tender.
5. Once cooked, remove the vegetables from the air fryer and set them to one side to cool down.
6. Transfer the vegetables to a food processor, add the lime juice so there are still chunks remaining.
7. Pour the salsa into a sealable jar and chill in the fridge before serving.

Hash Faux-Tato

Nutrition: Calories: 69, Protein: 1 g, Fats: 5 g, Carbs: 2 g, Fiber: 2 g

Total Time: 25 minutes

Servings: 4

Ingredients:

- ¼ tsp of black pepper
- ½ tsp of garlic powder
- 2 tbsp of melted butter
- ½ a medium green bell pepper, chopped and seeds removed
- ¼ of a diced medium yellow onion
- ½ tsp of salt
- 1 lb (454 g) of radishes, ends cut off and quartered

Instructions:

1. Set the air fryer to 320° F (160 ° C).
2. Combine the onions, green peppers and radishes, and butter in a baking dish.
3. Toss with garlic powder, salt and black pepper.
4. Put the baking dish into the air fryer and cook for 12 minutes.
5. Shake the basket halfway through.
6. The vegetables will be tender when cooked.
7. Once cooked, remove the baking dish from the air fryer and serve.

Roasted Garlic-Parmesan Cauliflower

Nutrition: Calories: 94, Protein: 4 g, Fats: 6 g, Carbs: 4 g, Fiber: 2 g

Total Time: 25 minutes

Servings: 4

Ingredients:

- 1 oz (45 g) of Parmesan cheese, grated
- 2 cloves of finely chopped garlic
- ½ tbsp of salt
- 1 medium head of cauliflower cut into florets
- 2 tbsp of melted salted butter

Instructions:

1. Set the air fryer to 350° F (177° C).
2. Put the cauliflower into a baking dish and brush with the butter.
3. Add the garlic, salt, and half of the Parmesan cheese and toss to combine.
4. Put the baking dish in the air fryer and cook for 15 minutes.
5. Shake the basket halfway through.
6. The cauliflower is ready when it's tender and browned around the edges.
7. Once the cauliflower is cooked, serve with the remaining Parmesan cheese.

Asparagus Flavored With Thyme & Lemon

Nutrition: Calories: 103, Protein: 5 g, Fats: 7 g, Carbs: 7 g, Fiber: 3 g

Total Time: 15 minutes

Servings: 4

Ingredients:

- The juice and zest of 1 lemon
- 2 oz (57 g) of crumbled goat cheese
- Salt and pepper to taste
- ½ tsp of dried thyme
- 1 tbsp of avocado oil
- 1 lb (454 g) of asparagus, ends trimmed

Instructions:

1. Set the air fryer to 400° F (204° C).
2. Place the asparagus, avocado oil, goat cheese, thyme, juice, zest of lemon and a pinch of salt and pepper in a baking dish and toss to combine.
3. Put the baking dish in the air fryer and cook for 6 minutes.
4. Shake the basket halfway through.
5. The asparagus will be tender and golden brown when cooked.
6. Once cooked remove the baking dish from the air fryer and serve.

Brussels Sprouts and Bacon

Nutrition: Calories: 89, Protein: 11 g, Fats: 5 g, Carbs: 5 g, Fiber: 3 g

Total Time: 30 minutes

Servings: 6

Ingredients:

- 4 strips of cooked and crumbled bacon
- Salt and pepper to taste

- 1 tsp of smoked paprika
- 1 tsp of garlic powder
- 1 tbsp of coconut aminos
- 1 tbsp of avocado oil
- 1 lb (454 g) of Brussels sprouts, halved and trimmed

Instructions:

1. Set the air fryer to 375° F (190° C).
2. In a baking dish, combine the Brussels sprouts, smoke paprika, garlic powder, coconut aminos, avocado oil, season with salt and pepper and toss to combine.
3. Put the baking tray in the air fryer and cook for 15 minutes.
4. Shake the basket halfway through.
5. The Brussels sprouts are cooked once they become tender and golden brown in color.
6. Once cooked, remove the baking dish from the air fryer, toss with the cooked bacon and serve.

Garlic & Lemon Flavored Mushrooms

Nutrition: Calories: 80, Protein: 1 g, Fats: 8 g, Carbs: 1 g, Fiber: 0 g

Total Time: 20 minutes

Servings: 6

Ingredients:

- 2 tbsp of fresh, chopped parsley
- ½ tsp of red pepper flakes
- 1 tsp of freshly squeezed lemon juice
- 1 clove of finely chopped garlic
- 3 tbsp of unsalted butter
- Salt and pepper to taste
- 1 tbsp of avocado oil
- 12 oz (340 g) of sliced mushrooms

Instructions:

1. Set the air fryer to 375° F (190° C).
2. Add the mushrooms to a baking dish, brush with avocado oil and season with salt and pepper
3. Put the baking dish in the air fryer and cook for 15 minutes.
4. The mushrooms are cooked once they turn golden brown in color.
5. Heat a small frying pan and melt the butter.
6. Add the garlic and fry for 30 seconds.
7. Remove the frying pan from the heat, add the red pepper flakes and the lemon juice and stir to combine.
8. Once cooked, remove the baking dish from the air fryer.
9. Toss the mushrooms in the garlic butter mix, top with parsley and serve.

Buttered Green Beans

Nutrition: Calories: 134, Protein: 3 g, Fats: 11 g, Carbs: 3 g, Fiber: 3 g

Total Time: 15 minutes

Servings: 6

Ingredients:

- 1 lb (454 g) of trimmed green beans
- .8 oz (23 g) Parmesan cheese
- 2.1 oz (60 g) melted unsalted butter

- Salt and pepper to taste
- 1 tsp of garlic powder
- 1 tbsp of avocado oil

Instructions:

1. Set the air fryer to 400° F (204° C).
2. Add the green beans, avocado oil, garlic powder, salt and pepper to a large bowl and toss to combine.
3. Put the beans into the air fryer and cook for 10 minutes.
4. Shake the basket halfway through.
5. The beans will be slightly brown around the edges when cooked.
6. Once cooked, remove the beans from the air fryer and put them into a large bowl.
7. Toss with the melted butter, top with Parmesan cheese and serve.

Fried Green Tomatoes

Nutrition: Calories: 106, Protein: 6 g, Fats: 7 g, Carbs: 6 g, Fiber: 2 g

Total Time: 20 minutes

Servings: 4

Ingredients:

- 1 oz (30 g) of grated Parmesan cheese
- .8 oz (23 g) of blanched finely ground almond flour
- 1 large egg
- 2 medium green tomatoes cut into ½ inch thick slices

Instructions:

1. Set the air fryer to 400° F (204° C).
2. Whisk the egg in a medium sized bowl.
3. In a large bowl, add the Parmesan cheese and the almond flour and toss to combine.
4. One at a time, dip the tomatoes into the egg and then into the flour mixture.
5. Put the tomatoes into the air fryer and cook for 7 minutes.
6. Flip the tomatoes halfway through.
7. The tomatoes will be golden brown in color when cooked.
8. Once cooked, remove the tomatoes from the air fryer and serve.

Asparagus Wrapped in Bacon

Nutrition: Calories: 110, Protein: 8 g, Fats: 7 g, Carbs: 3 g, Fiber: 2 g

Total Time: 20 minutes

Servings: 4

Ingredients:

- 1 lb (453 g) of asparagus spears, woody ends trimmed
- 8 slices of bacon cut in halves

Instructions:

1. Set the air fryer to 350° F (177° C).
2. Wrap 1 piece of bacon around the middle of each asparagus.
3. Put the asparagus into the air fryer and cook for 10 minutes.
4. When the bacon turns crispy and golden brown in color, they're cooked.

5. Once cooked, remove the asparagus from the air fryer and serve.

Chapter 9: Vegetarian Mains

Discover loads of colorful and fresh vegetarian main course recipes from tangy sweet & spicy nachos to heart-warming Italian style vegetables and more.

Spaghetti Alfredo

Nutrition: Calories: 375, Protein: 13 g, Fats: 24 g, Carbs: 20 g, Fiber: 4 g

Total Time: 25 minutes

Servings: 2

Ingredients:

- 1 oz (45 g) shredded Italian blend cheese
- ¼ tsp of ground peppercorn
- 1 tsp of dried parsley
- ½ tsp of garlic powder
- .8 oz (23 g) vegetarian Parmesan cheese, grated
- 4 oz (113 g) of low-carb Alfredo sauce
- 2 tbsp of salted melted butter
- ½ a large cooked spaghetti squash

Instructions:

1. Set the air fryer to 320° F (160° C).
2. Scrape the spaghetti squash threads out with a fork.
3. In a medium sized bowl, combine the Alfredo sauce and the butter and stir together thoroughly.
4. Add the Parmesan cheese, parsley, garlic powder, Italian blend cheese and ground peppercorn and stir to combine.
5. Pour the mixture into a 4-cup round baking dish.
6. Put the baking dish in the microwave and cook for 15 minutes.
7. The cheese will be golden brown in color and bubbling when cooked.
8. Once cooked, remove the baking dish from the air fryer and serve.

Cabbage Crispy Steaks

Nutrition: Calories: 105, Protein: 2 g, Fats: 7 g, Carbs: 6 g, Fiber: 5 g

Total Time: 15 minutes

Servings: 4

Ingredients:

- 1 small cabbage head, core removed and cut into slices ½ an inch thick
- 1 clove of finely chopped garlic
- 2 tbsp of olive oil
- ¼ tsp of ground black pepper
- ¼ tsp of salt

Instructions:

1. Set the air fryer to 350° F (177° C).
2. Season the cabbage with chopped garlic , salt and pepper.
3. Drizzle olive oil over the cabbage.
4. Grease the air fryer basket and add the cabbage.
5. Cook the cabbage steaks for 10 minutes.
6. Turn the cabbage steaks after 5 minutes.
7. When the cabbage steaks are ready, they will be tender all

the way through, and the outer edges will be golden brown in color.

Sweet & Spicy Nachos

Nutrition: Calories: 310, Protein: 12 g, Fats: 23 g, Carbs: 11 g, Fiber: 5 g

Total Time: 15 minutes

Servings: 2

Ingredients:

- 2 tbsp of sour cream
- ½ a medium avocado, peeled, seed removed and diced
- 2 oz (57 g) pickled jalapenos, sliced
- 2.4 oz (68 g) of Colby Jack Cheese, shredded
- 6 small, sweet peppers, seeds removed and cut in half

Instructions:

1. Set the air fryer to 350° F (177° C).
2. Arrange the peppers in a non-stick baking dish.
3. Sprinkle with the cheese and jalapenos.
4. Put the dish into the air fryer and cook for 5 minutes.
5. The cheese is ready when it's bubbly and melted.
6. Serve with avocado and a dollop of sour cream.

Italian Style Veg With Baked Eggs

Nutrition: Calories: 150, Protein: 8 g, Fats: 10 g, Carbs: 6 g, Fiber: 2 g

Total Time: 20 minutes

Servings: 2

Ingredients:

- 1 diced medium Roma tomato
- 1 oz (30g) chopped fresh spinach
- ½ a medium green bell pepper, diced and seeds removed
- 1 small zucchini, sliced into quarters
- ¼ tsp of dried oregano
- ½ tsp of dried basil
- ¼ tsp of onion powder
- 2 large eggs
- ¼ tsp of salt
- 2 tbsp of salted butter

Instructions:

1. Set the air fryer to 330° F(166° C).
2. Grease two ramekins with 2 spoonful of butter each.
3. In a large bowl, combine the tomatoes, spinach, bell pepper, and zucchini and toss to combine.
4. Transfer ¼ of the vegetable mix into one ramekin.
5. Transfer ½ of the vegetable mix into the other ramekin.

6. Add eggs over each ramekin.

7. Season both ramekins with oregano, basil, salt and onion powder.

8. Put the ramekins into the air fryer and cook for 10 minutes.

9. Once cooked, remove from the air fryer and serve.

Parmesan Flavored Artichokes

Nutrition: Calories: 189, Protein: 8 g, Fats: 13 g, Carbs: 10 g, Fiber: 4 g

Total Time: 20 minutes

Servings: 4

Ingredients:

- ½ tsp of crushed pepper flakes
- .8 oz (23 g) blanched almond flour, finely ground
- 1 oz (45 g) of vegetarian Parmesan cheese, grated
- 1 whisked large egg
- 2 tbsp of olive oil
- ¼ tsp of salt
- 2 medium artichokes, middle removed, quartered and trimmed

Instructions:

1. Set the air fryer to 400° F (204° C).

2. Place the artichokes into a large bowl and toss with the olive oil and salt.

3. In a large bowl, add the Parmesan cheese and almond flour and toss to combine.

4. Dip 1 piece of artichoke into the egg at a time and then dip into the almond flour mix.

5. Sprinkle with the pepper flakes.

6. Arrange the artichokes in the air fryer and cook for 10 minutes.

7. Toss the artichokes halfway through.

8. Once cooked, remove from the air fryer and serve.

Roasted Lemon Flavored Cauliflower

Nutrition: Calories: 91, Protein: 3 g, Fats: 6 g, Carbs: 5 g, Fiber: 3 g

Total Time: 20 minutes

Servings: 4

Ingredients:

- 1 medium cauliflower head, sliced into florets
- 1 tsp of dried parsley
- ½ tsp of garlic powder
- The juice from 1 medium lemon
- The zest from ½ a medium lemon
- 2 tbsp of melted salted butter
- ¼ tsp of salt

Instructions:

1. Set the air fryer to 350° F (177° C).

2. Put the cauliflower florets into a large bowl and brush with melted butter.

3. Add the lemon zest.

4. Drizzle the lemon juice over the top and toss to combine.

5. Add the parsley and toss to combine.

6. Add the garlic powder , salt and toss to combine.

7. Transfer the cauliflower into the air fryer and cook for 15 minutes.

8. Once cooked, remove from the air fryer and serve.

Greek Style Stuffed Eggplant

Nutrition: Calories: 291, Protein: 9 g, Fats: 19 g, Carbs: 12 g, Fiber: 11 g

Total Time: 35 minutes

Servings:

Ingredients:

- 1 large eggplant, sliced lengthwise, dice the middle
- 1 oz (45 g) of crumbled feta cheese
- 2 tbsp of diced red bell pepper
- 1 oz (30 g) of fresh spinach
- 2 oz (57 g) of artichoke hearts, chopped
- ¼ of a medium yellow onion, diced
- 2 tbsp of unsalted butter

Instructions:

1. Set the air fryer to 320° F (160° C).

2. Heat the butter in a medium sized frying pan and cook the onions for 3 minutes.

3. Add the bell peppers, spinach, and artichoke hearts, stir to combine and cook for 5 minutes.

4. Remove the frying pan from the stove, add the feta cheese and toss to combine.

5. Spoon the cooked mixture into the eggplant boats.

6. Put the eggplant boats into the air fryer and cook for 20 minutes.

7. Once the eggplants are tender, remove them from the air fryer and serve.

Bowl of Roasted Veggies

Nutrition: Calories: 121, Protein: 4 g, Fats: 7 g, Carbs: 13 g, Fiber: 5 g

Total Time: 25 minutes

Servings: 2

Ingredients:

- ½ a medium bell pepper, seeds removed and sliced into ¼ of an inch pieces
- ¼ medium white onion, peeled and sliced into ¼ inch pieces
- 4 oz (113 g) of cauliflower florets
- 2.5 oz (70 g) Brussels sprouts, quartered
- 2.5 oz (70 g) broccoli florets
- 1 tbsp of coconut oil
- ½ tsp of cumin
- ½ tsp of garlic powder
- 2 tsp of chili powder

Instructions:

1. Set the air fryer to 360° F (182° C).

2. In a large bowl, add all the ingredients and toss to combine.

3. Transfer the vegetables to the air fryer and cook for 15 minutes.

4. Toss the basket halfway through.

5. Once cooked, remove the vegetables from the air fryer and serve.

Mini Portobello Pizzas

Nutrition: Calories: 244, Protein: 10 g, Fats: 18 g, Carbs: 7 g, Fiber: 2 g

Total Time: 20 minutes

Servings: 2

Ingredients:

- 2 large Portobello mushrooms, stems removed
- 1 tbsp of balsamic vinegar
- 2 leaves of fresh basil, chopped
- 4 sliced grape tomatoes
- 5.3 oz (150 g) of Mozzarella cheese, shredded
- ½ tsp of garlic powder
- 2 tbsp of melted unsalted butter

Instructions:

1. Set the air fryer to 380° F (193° C).
2. Smear butter over the mushrooms and sprinkle with garlic powder.
3. Put some tomatoes and cheese into the base of the mushrooms.
4. Put the mushrooms onto a non-stick baking pan.
5. Put the baking pan into the air fryer and cook for 10 minutes.
6. Once the mushrooms are cooked, remove them from the air fryer.
7. Drizzle with balsamic vinegar, sprinkle the basil leaves over the top and serve.

Cheesy Zucchini Boats

Nutrition: Calories: 215, Protein: 10 g, Fats: 15 g, Carbs: 9 g, Fiber: 3 g

Total Time: 35 minutes

Servings: 2

Ingredients:

- 2 medium zucchinis, ends chopped off, sliced in half and middle scooped out
- 2 tbsp of vegetarian Parmesan cheese
- ½ tsp of dried parsley
- ¼ tsp of garlic powder
- ¼ tsp of dried oregano
- .8 oz (23 g) Mozzarella cheese, shredded
- .8 oz (23 g) of ricotta cheese, full fat
- 4 oz (113 g) pasta sauce, no added sugar and low carb
- 1 tbsp of avocado oil

Instructions:

1. Set the air fryer to 350° F (177° C).
2. Grease the zucchini boats with avocado oil.
3. Fill each boat with 2 tablespoons of pasta sauce.
4. Add the Mozzarella cheese, ricotta cheese, parsley, garlic powder and oregano to a large bowl and toss to combine.
5. Spoon the mixture into the boats.
6. Place the zucchini boats into the air fryer and cook for 20 minutes.

7. Once cooked, remove the zucchini boats from the air fryer, sprinkle with Parmesan cheese and serve.

Vegetable Burgers

Nutrition: Calories: 48, Protein: 3 g, Fats: 2 g, Carbs: 5 g, Fiber: 1 g

Total Time: 12 minutes

Servings: 4

Ingredients:

- ¼ tsp of ground black pepper
- ½ tsp of salt
- 1 clove of finely chopped garlic
- 2 oz (57 g) of chopped yellow onion
- ½ a medium zucchini, chopped and trimmed
- 2 large egg yolks
- 8 oz (113 g) of cremini mushrooms

Instructions:

1. Set the air fryer to 375° F (190° C).
2. Put all the ingredients into a food processor and pulse until combined.
3. Create four patties out of the mixture.
4. Put the patties into the air fryer and cook for 12 minutes.
5. The patties will be golden brown in color when cooked.
6. Once the patties are cooked, remove them from the air fryer and serve.

Peppers Stuffed With Cauliflower Rice

Nutrition: Calories: 185, Protein: 9 g, Fats: 12 g, Carbs: 11 g, Fiber: 4 g

Total Time: 15 minutes

Servings: 4

Ingredients:

- 4 medium bell peppers, seeded and tops removed
- ¼ tsp of ground black pepper
- ¼ tsp of salt
- 8 oz (227 g) of Mozzarella cheese, shredded
- 2 tbsp of olive oil
- 5.3 oz (150 g) of canned, diced tomatoes, drained
- 7 oz (200 g) of uncooked cauliflower rice

Instructions:

1. Set the air fryer to 350° F (177° C).
2. Combine all the ingredients (except the bell peppers) in a large bowl and stir to combine.
3. Spoon the mixture into the bell peppers.
4. Place the bell peppers in the air fryer and cook for 15 minutes.
5. The peppers are cooked when they become tender, and the cheese has melted.
6. Once cooked, remove the bell peppers from the air fryer and serve.

Pizza With Broccoli Base

Nutrition: Calories: 136, Protein: 10 g, Fats: 7 g, Carbs: 4 g, Fiber: 2 g

Total Time: 30 minutes

Servings: 4

Ingredients:

- 1 oz (45 g) of shredded Mozzarella cheese
- 3 tbsp of low-carb Alfredo sauce
- 1 oz (45 g) of vegetarian Parmesan cheese, grated
- 1 large egg
- ¼ tsp of salt
- 10 oz (300 g) of rice broccoli, steamed and drained

Instructions:

1. Set the air fryer to 370° F (188° C).
2. Combine the Parmesan cheese, salt , egg, and broccoli in a large bowl and stir together thoroughly.
3. Lay a sheet of parchment paper in the air fryer basket.
4. Spread the pizza crust mixture on top of the parchment paper.
5. Cook the pizza crust for 7 minutes.
6. Flip the pizza crust and top with Alfredo sauce and Mozzarella and cook for another 7 minutes.
7. The pizza is cooked when the cheese is bubbling and golden brown in color.
8. Once cooked, remove the pizza from the air fryer and serve.

Cheesy Spinach Pie

Nutrition: Calories: 288, Protein: 18 g, Fats: 20 g, Carbs: 2 g, Fiber: 2 g

Total Time: 30 minutes

Servings: 4

Ingredients:

- 2 oz (57 g) of yellow onion, diced
- 4 oz (113 g) sharp cheddar cheese, shredded
- 1 oz (30 g), chopped spinach
- 2 oz (57 g) of heavy whipping cream
- ¼ tsp of salt
- 6 large eggs

Instructions:

1. Set the air fryer to 320° F (160 ° C).
2. Add the cream, salt and eggs to a medium bowl and whisk to combine.
3. Add the spinach, cheese, and onions and whisk to combine.
4. Pour the batter into a 9-inch round baking dish.
5. Put the baking dish into the air fryer and cook for 20 minutes.
6. When cooked, the eggs will slightly browned and firm.
7. Remove the pie from the air fryer and serve.

Chapter 10: Delicious Desserts

Discover delightful desserts for all occasions. These recipes are quick and easy to make but taste like something out of a 5-star restaurant.

Protein Powder Doughnuts

Nutrition: Calories: 221, Protein: 20 g, Fats: 1 g, Carbs: 4 g, Fiber: 2 g

Total Time: 50 minutes

Servings: 12 doughnuts (3 per person)

Ingredients:

- ½ tsp of vanilla extract
- 5 tbsp of melted unsalted butter
- 1 large egg
- ½ tsp of baking powder
- 3.7 oz (105 g) of granulated erythritol
- 1 oz (30 g) of low-carb vanilla protein powder
- 2 oz (60 g) of blanched finely ground almond powder

Instructions:

1. Set the air fryer to 380° F (193° C).
2. Put all the ingredients into a large bowl, stir to combine and put the bowl in the fridge for 20 minutes.
3. Remove the batter from the fridge, knead the dough and create 12 dough balls.
4. Place a sheet of parchment paper into the air fryer basket.
5. Arrange the dough balls in the air fryer and cook for 6 minutes.
6. Turn the doughnuts after 3 minutes.
7. Once cooked, remove the doughnuts from the air fryer and leave them to cool down before serving.

Chocolate Chip Cookies

Nutrition: Calories: 188, Protein: 5 g, Fats: 16 g, Carbs: 4 g, Fiber: 2 g

Total Time: 20 minutes

Servings: 4

Ingredients:

- 2 tbsp of sugar-free, low-carb chocolate chips
- ½ tsp of vanilla extract
- ½ tsp of baking powder
- ½ tsp of unflavored gelatine
- 1 large egg
- 2 tbsp of softened, unsalted butter
- 1 oz (45 g) of erythritol
- 2.1 oz (60 g) of blanched finely ground almond flour

Instructions:

1. Set the air-fryer to 300° F (149° C).
2. In a large bowl, add the erythritol and flour and stir to combine.
3. Add the gelatine, egg, and butter, and stir to combine.
4. Add the vanilla and the baking powder and stir to combine.
5. Add the chocolate chips and stir to combine.
6. Spoon the batter into a 9-inch pie plate.

7. Put the plate into the air fryer and cook for 7 minutes.
8. Pierce the cookie with a toothpick, if it comes out clean, it's cooked.
9. Once cooked, remove the cookie from the air fryer, leave it to cool down for 10 minutes before serving.

Macademia Nut Brownies

Nutrition: Calories: 112, Protein: 2 g, Fats: 8 g, Carbs: 8 g, Fiber: 3 g

Total Time: 35 minutes

Servings: 12 brownies (3 per person)

Ingredients:

- 2 oz (45 g) of crushed macadamia nuts
- 1 egg
- 4 oz (113 g) of melted dark chocolate
- 1 tsp of fresh lemon juice
- ½ tsp of baking powder
- 3 oz (87 g) of coconut flour
- 3 tbsp of melted butter

Instructions:

1. Set the air fryer to 355° F (179° C).
2. In a large bowl, add the egg and melted butter and whisk to combine.
3. Add the melted dark chocolate, lemon juice, baking powder, and coconut flour and whisk to combine.
4. Add the macadamia nuts and stir to combine.
5. Spoon the brownie dough into a 9-inch round baking pan.
6. Put the baking pan in the air fryer and cook for 25 minutes.
7. When the dough turns golden brown in color, it's ready.
8. Remove the baking tray from the air fryer and leave it to cool down completely before slicing and serving.

Walnut Flavored Cheesecake

Nutrition: Calories: 531, Protein: 11 g, Fats: 7 g, Carbs: 5 g, Fiber: 2 g

Total Time: 20 minutes

Servings: 4

Ingredients:

- 8 oz (23 g) of powdered erythritol
- ½ tsp of vanilla extract
- 1 large egg
- 4 oz (113 g) of softened full-fat cream cheese
- 2 tbsp of granulated erythritol
- 2 tbsp of salted butter
- 2 oz (56 g) of walnuts

Instructions:

1. Set the air fryer to 400° F (204° C).
2. Make a dough by putting the walnuts, granulated erythritol

and butter into a food processor and blend to combine.

3. Transfer the dough into a spring foam pan and spread out to fill the pan.

4. Put the pan in the air fryer and cook for five minutes.

5. Remove the pan from the air fryer and put it to one side.

6. In a medium sized bowl, combine the egg, powdered erythritol, vanilla extract and cream cheese.

7. Spread the mixture over the walnut crust.

8. Turn the air fryer down to 300° F (149° C).

9. Put the pan back into the air fryer and cook for ten minutes.

10. Once cooked, remove the cheesecake from the air fryer, leave it to cool completely to room temperature, and then put it in the fridge to chill before serving.

Almond Butter Flavored Cookie Balls

Nutrition: Calories: 224, Protein: 11 g, Fats: 16 g, Carbs: 6 g, Fiber: 4 g

Total Time: 15 minutes

Servings: 8 cookie balls (2 per person)

Ingredients:

- ½ tsp of ground cinnamon
- 1.4 oz (40 g) of sugar-free, low-carb chocolate chips
- .6 oz (18 g) shredded coconut, unsweetened
- .8 oz (45 g) of powered erythritol
- ¾ oz (21 g) of protein powder, low carb
- 1 tsp of vanilla extract
- 1 large egg
- 8 oz (227 g) of almond butter

Instructions:

1. Set the air fryer to 320° F(160° C)

2. In a large bowl, combine the almond butter, vanilla extract, erythritol, egg, and protein powder and whisk to combine.

3. Add the coconut, cinnamon, and chocolate chip cookies and stir to combine.

4. Divide the dough into 8 balls and arrange them in the air fryer.

5. Cook for 10 minutes.

6. Once cooked, remove the cookie balls from the air fryer and leave to cool down completely before serving.

Blackberry Tart

Nutrition: Calories: 78, Protein: 2 g, Fats: 7 g, Carbs: 8 g, Fiber: 1 g

Total Time: 45 minutes

Servings: 12 Tarts (3 per person)

Ingredients:

- 1 egg
- 2 tbsp of coconut flour
- 1 tsp of vanilla extract
- 1 pinch of salt
- 4 tbsp of butter
- 3.4 oz (96 g) almond flour
- 2 oz (58 g) of erythritol
- 2 oz (71 g) blackberry

Instructions:

1. Set the air fryer to 355° F (179° C).

2. In a large bowl, combine the blackberries and erythritol, stir to combine and put it to one side.

3. In another large bowl add the egg and whisk together thoroughly.

4. Add the almond flour and salt and whisk to combine.

5. Add the coconut flour, butter, and vanilla extract and whisk to combine.

6. Knead the dough on a flat surface and roll it out.

7. Place a sheet of parchment paper in the air fryer.

8. Put the rolled dough in the air fryer.

9. Spoon the blackberry mixture on top of the dough.

10. Cook the tart for 25 minutes.

11. The dough will become golden brown in color when the tart is cooked.

12. Once the tart is cooked, remove it from the air fryer, and leave it to cool down completely before serving.

Luscious Lime Bars

Nutrition: Calories: 133, Protein: 4 g, Fats: 12 g, Carbs: 3 g, Fiber: 1 g

Total Time: 45 minutes

Servings: 12 bars (3 per person)

Ingredients:

- 2 large eggs, whisked
- 4 oz (113 g) of fresh lime juice
- 4 tbsp of melted salted butter
- .8 oz (45 g) of powdered erythritol
- 5 oz (144 g) of blanched finely ground almond flour

Instructions:

1. Set the air fryer to 300° F (149° C).

2. In a medium sized bowl, combine the flour, butter, and erythritol and whisk to combine.

3. Transfer the mixture into a 9-inch round baking pan.

4. Put the baking pan into the air fryer and cook for 13 minutes.

5. The crust will be a golden-brown color once cooked.

6. Remove the crust from the air fryer and leave it to cool down completely.

7. Combine the remaining flour, and erythritol, eggs, and lime juice into a medium sized bowl and stir together thoroughly.

8. Spoon the mixture over the top of the cooled crust and cook for 20 minutes on 300° F.

9. The top will be firm and browned once cooked.

10. Remove the pan from the air fryer and leave to cool down completely.

11. Once cooled, slice into bars and place in the fridge to chill before serving.

Shortbread Cream Cheese Cookies

Nutrition: Calories: 175, Protein: 5 g, Fats: 16 g, Carbs: 2 g, Fiber: 2 g

Total Time: 50 minutes

Servings: 12 cookies (3 per person)

Ingredients:

- 1 tsp of almond extract
- 6 oz (192 g) blanched finely ground almond flour

- 1 large egg
- 3 oz (100 g) of granulated erythritol
- 2 oz (57 g) of softened cream cheese
- 2 oz (57 g) of melted coconut oil

Instructions:

1. Set the air fryer to 320° F (160° C).
2. Add all the ingredients to a large bowl and whisk to combine.
3. Roll the dough into a 12-inch log and place it onto a sheet of plastic wrap.
4. Wrap the dough up with the plastic wrap and place it in the fridge to chill for 30 minutes.
5. Remove the dough from the fridge and slice it into 12 even cookies.
6. Line the air fryer basket with parchment paper.
7. Arrange the cookies in the air fryer basket and cook for 10 minutes.
8. Flip the cookies after 5 minutes.
9. The cookies will be golden brown in color when cooked.
10. Remove the cookies from the air fryer and leave to cool down completely before serving.

Strawberry Shortcake

Nutrition: Calories: 235, Protein: 6 g, Fats: 21 g, Carbs: 3 g, Fiber: 2 g

Total Time: 35 minutes

Servings: 6

Ingredients:

- 6 medium sized fresh strawberries, sliced and hulled
- 17 oz (480 g) of whipped-cream, sugar-free
- 1 tsp of vanilla extract
- 1 tsp of baking powder
- 3 oz (100 g) granulated erythritol
- 2 large eggs
- 3 oz (96 g) blanched finely ground almond flour
- 2 tbsp of coconut oil

Instructions:

1. Set the air fryer to 300° F (149° C).
2. In a large bowl, add all the ingredients and whisk to combine.
3. Pour the batter into a 9-inch round baking dish.
4. Place the baking dish into the air fryer and cook for 25 minutes.
5. The shortcake will be golden brown in color when cooked.
6. Remove the shortcake from the air fryer and leave it to cool down completely before serving.

Chocolate Brownies

Nutrition: Calories: 367, Protein: 14 g, Fats: 32 g, Carbs: 5 g, Fiber: 4 g

Total Time: 35 minutes

Servings: 2

Ingredients:

- 4 oz (123 g) sour cream
- 1 tsp of vanilla extract
- 1 tsp of baking powder

- 3 oz (100 g) granulated erythritol
- 2 large eggs
- 1.1 oz (32 g) coconut flour
- 2 tbsp of melted salted butter
- Cooking oil spray

Instructions:

1. Set the air fryer to 300° F (149° C).
2. Add all the ingredients to a large bowl and whisk to combine.
3. Lightly spray two ramekins with cooking oil.
4. Spoon the batter into the ramekins and place them into the air fryer.
5. Cook the brownies for 15 minutes.
6. Once cooked, the middle of the brownies will be firm.
7. Remove the brownies from the air fryer and leave them to cool down for completely before serving.

Coconut Cake

Nutrition: Calories: 367, Protein: 14 g, Fats: 32 g, Carbs: 5 g, Fiber: 4 g

Total Time: 35 minutes

Servings: 6

Ingredients:

- 4.3 oz (123 g) of sour cream
- 1 tsp of vanilla extract
- 1 tsp of baking powder
- 3.1 oz (90 g) of granulated erythritol
- 2 large eggs
- 1.1 oz (32 g) coconut flour
- 2 tbsp of melted salted butter

Instructions:

1. Set the air fryer to 300° F (149° C).
2. Add all the ingredients into a large bowl and whisk to combine.
3. Pour the batter into a 9-inch round baking dish.
4. The cake will be a deep golden color when cooked, you should also be able to stick a toothpick in the middle and it should have nothing on it when you pull it out.
5. Remove the cake from the air fryer and leave it to cool down completely before serving.

Clustered Pecans

Nutrition: Calories: 136, Protein: 2 g, Fats: 9 g, Carbs: 11 g, Fiber: 9 g

Total Time: 20 minutes

Servings: 2

Ingredients:

- 5 oz (150 g) of low-carb chocolate chips
- ½ tsp of ground cinnamon
- 3 oz (85 g) of whole shelled pecans
- 3 tbsp of granulated erythritol

Instructions:

1. Set the air fryer to 350° F (177° C).
2. In a medium sized bowl, combine the pecans, cinnamon, and

erythritol.

3. Transfer the pecan mixture to a baking dish.

4. Put the baking dish into the air fryer and cook for 8 minutes.

5. Once the pecans are cooked, remove them from the air fryer and put them to one side.

6. Shake the basket halfway through.

7. Place a sheet of parchment paper over a large baking sheet.

8. Put the chocolate chips into a medium sized microwavable bowl and melt until smooth.

9. Arrange the pecans on the baking sheet in clusters.

10. Pour the melted chocolate over each pecan cluster.

11. Put the baking sheet in the fridge and leave it to set for 30 minutes.

12. Once set, remove the baking sheet from the fridge and serve.

Lava Chocolate Cake

Nutrition: Calories: 282, Protein: 9 g, Fats: 23 g, Carbs: 13 g, Fiber: 10 g

Total Time: 20 minutes

Servings: 2

Ingredients:

- 2 oz (57 g) of low-carb chocolate chips
- ½ tsp of vanilla extract
- .8 oz (24 g) blanched finely ground almond flour
- 2 large eggs
- Cooking spray

Instructions:

1. Set the air fryer to 320° F (160° C).

2. Place the chocolate chips into a microwavable bowl and melt.

3. Combine all the ingredients (including the melted chocolate) into a large bowl and whisk.

4. Lightly spray two ramekins with cooking spray.

5. Spoon the cake mixture into the ramekins.

6. Put the ramekins into the air fryer and cook for 15 minutes.

7. The cake will be set around the edges and firm in the middle once cooked.

8. Remove the ramekins from the air fryer and leave to cool down completely before serving.

Peanut Butter Crustless Cheesecake

Nutrition: Calories: 282, Protein: 9 g, Fats: 23 g, Carbs: 13 g, Fiber: 10 g

Total Time: 20 minutes

Servings: 2

Ingredients:

- 1 large egg
- ½ tsp of vanilla extract
- 1 tbsp of sugar-free peanut butter
- 2 tbsp of granulated erythritol
- 4 oz (113 g) of softened cream cheese

Instructions:

1. Set the air fryer to 300° F (149° C)

2. In a large bowl, combine all the ingredients and whisk.

3. Transfer the mixture into a spring foam pan and spread out evenly.

4. Put the pan into the air fryer and cook for 10 minutes.

5. The cheesecake will be slightly firm.

6. Remove the cheesecake from the air fryer and leave it to cool down completely.

7. Once the cheesecake has cooled down, put it in the fridge to chill before serving.

8. Once chilled, remove from the fridge and serve.

Danish Cream Cheese

Nutrition: Calories: 185, Protein: 7 g, Fats: 14 g, Carbs: 9 g, Fiber: 2 g

Total Time: 35 minutes

Servings: 6

Ingredients:

- 2 tsp of vanilla extract
- 2.4 oz (68 g) of powdered erythritol
- 2 large egg yolks
- 5 oz (142 g) of full-fat cream cheese
- 3.1 oz (90 g) shredded Mozzarella cheese
- 2 oz (72 g) blanched finely ground almond flour

Instructions:

1. Place a sheet of parchment paper in the air fryer basket.

2. In a large microwave safe bowl, add the half the cream cheese, Mozzarella, almond flour, stir to combine and microwave for 1 minute.

3. Remove the bowl from the microwave, add the egg yolks and stir to combine.

4. Add the half the erythritol and 1 teaspoon of vanilla extract and stir to combine.

5. Knead out the dough into a ¼ inch thick rectangle.

6. In a medium sized bowl, add the rest of the cream cheese, erythritol and vanilla and stir to combine.

7. Spoon the cream cheese mixture out onto the right half of the dough and fold the left half over it and seal the ends by pressing the dough together.

8. Set the air fryer to 330° F (166 ° C).

9. Put the Danish into the air fryer and cook for 15 minutes,

10. Flip the dough halfway through.

11. The Danish will be golden brown in color when cooked.

12. Once the Danish is cooked, remove it from the air fryer and leave it to cool down completely before serving.

Vanilla Pound Cake

Nutrition: Calories: 253, Protein: 7 g, Fats: 23 g, Carbs: 3 g, Fiber: 2 g

Total Time: 35 minutes

Servings: 6

Ingredients:

- 2 large eggs
- 1 oz (28 g) of softened full-fat cream cheese
- 4.3 oz (122 g) full fat sour cream
- 1 tsp of baking powder
- 1 tsp of vanilla extract
- 3.1 oz (90 g) granulated erythritol
- 2.1 oz (60 g) melted salted butter
- 3.3 oz (96 g) of blanched finely ground almond flour

Instructions:

1. Set the air fryer to 300° F (149° C).
2. Add the erythritol, butter, and almond flour to a large bowl and stir to combine.
3. Add the eggs and whisk to combine.
4. Add the cream cheese, sour cream, vanilla, and baking powder and whisk to combine.
5. Pour the batter into a 9-inch round baking pan.
6. Put the baking pan in the air fryer and let it cook for 25 minutes.
7. To check whether the cake is cooked, poke the middle all the way through with a toothpick, it's ready if the toothpick comes out clean.
8. Once cooked, remove the baking pan from the air fryer and leave the cake to cool down completely before serving.

Coconut Flavored Mug Cake

Nutrition: Calories: 237, Protein: 9 g, Fats: 16 g, Carbs: 10 g, Fiber: 5 g

Total Time: 30 minutes

Servings: 1

Ingredients:

- ¼ tsp of baking powder
- ¼ tsp of vanilla extract
- 2 tbsp of granulated erythritol
- 2 tbsp of heavy whipped cream
- 2 tbsp of coconut flour
- 2 large egg

Instructions:

1. Set the air fryer to 300° F (149° C).
2. Whisk the eggs in a 4-inch ramekin.
3. Add the rest of the ingredients and whisk until a smooth batter is formed.
4. Put the ramekin into the air fryer and cook for 25 minutes.
5. To check whether the cake is cooked, poke the middle all the way through with a toothpick. It's ready if the toothpick comes out clean.
6. Remove the cake out of the air fryer and serve.

Meal Plan Week 1

Day	Breakfast	Lunch	Snack	Dinner
Monday	Egg, Cheese and Spinach Omelette pg.21	Chicken Nuggets with Cheese pg.29	Crunchy Spinach Chips pg.28	Turkey Pot Pie pg.35
Tuesday	Peppers with Sausage pg.21	Cheese burger on a Stick pg.29	Parmesan Bell Pepper pg.28	Seasoned Rack of Lamb pg.41
Wednesday	Tomato Egg and Spinach pg.21	Pork Meatballs Pg.29	Bacon and Zucchini Cake pg.28	Spicy Chicken pg.35
Thursday	Almond Pecan Granola pg.22	Roasted Zucchini pg.30	Tomato Cheesy Flavored Chips pg.28	Cajun Flavored Haddock pg.48
Friday	Pepper and Ham Omelette pg. 21	Succulent Seasoned Eggplant pg.30	Crispy Cauliflower pg.29	Lamb Kebobs with Coconut Curry pg.41
Saturday	Breakfast lemon Cake pg. 22	BBQ Chicken Kebabs pg.35	French Fried Broccoli with Spicy Dip pg.30	Cod Sticks with Tartar Sauce pg.49
Sunday	Sausage Egg Cup pg. 22	Taco Rolls with Ground Beef pg.41	Kale Chips pg.30	Bacon with Tomato pg. 36

Meal Plan Week 2

Day	Breakfast	Lunch	Snack	Dinner
Monday	Egg Pepperoni pg. 22	Cheesy Vegetable Chicken pg.36	Golden Brussel Sprouts pg.30	Beef Tenderloin Encrusted with Peppercorns pg.42
Tuesday	Golden Muffins pg. 23	Beef Stir Fry with Broccoli pg.42	Pork Belly Flavored Chips pg.31	Sweet & Crisp Duck Legs pg.36
Wednesday	Ham and Avocado Delight pg. 23	Pork Meatballs pg.43	Cheesy Pickle Spear pg.31	Garlic Buttered Crab Legs pg.48
Thursday	Hash Brown Cauliflower pg. 24	Avocado Boats Stuffed with Crab pg.47	Crunchy Pepperoni Chips pg.31	Chicken and Bacon with Cheese pg.36
Friday	Cheddar Cheese Egg pg. 23	Cauliflower Chicken pg.37	Avocado French Fries pg.31	Shrimp Flavored with Lime and Chili pg.47
Saturday	Chocolate Chip Muffin pg.24	Cheesy Tuna Stuffed in Tomatoes pg.49	Crunchy Salami Cheese Roll-ups pg.32	Baby Spareribs pg.42
Sunday	Broccoli Fritatta pg.24	Taco Rolls with Ground Beef pg.41	Zucchini Cheesy Fries pg.32	Piri Piri Flavored Chicken Wings pg.39

Meal Plan Week 3

Day	Breakfast	Lunch	Snack	Dinner
Monday	Blueberry Muffins pg.24	Cheesy Chicken and Pork pg.32	Cauliflower Bacon Skewers pg.32	Chicken and Brussel Sprouts pg.39
Tuesday	Turkey Sausage pg.24	Chicken Wings and Eggs pg.33	Pork Rind Cheesy Tortillas pg.33	Cajun Salmon Patties pg.46
Wednesday	Pork Sausage Egg with Mustard Sauce Pg. 25	Golden Egg Pork pg.33	Crunchy Pepperoni Chips pg.31	Lamb Chops with Mojito Marinade pg.42
Thursday	Mushroom frittata pg.25	Cheesy Chicken Wings pg.33	Bacon and Zucchini Cheese Cake pg.28	Chicken and Ham with Cheese pg.40
Friday	Tomato and Mushroom Medley pg.25	Turkey Pot Pie pg.35	Crispy Cauliflower pg.29	Stuffed Flounder Florentine pg.46
Saturday	Aromatic Cake pg.26	Pork Meatballs pg.43	Kale Chips pg.30	Creamy Chicken pg.38
Sunday	Egg Bacon Cheese and Avocado pg.25	Crunchy Salami Cheese Roll-Ups pg.32	French Fry Styled Broccoli With Spicy Dip pg.30	Catfish Encrusted with Pecans pg.47

Day	Breakfast	Lunch	Snack	Dinner
Monday	Cheese and Bacon Flatbread pg.26	Sweet and Sour Pork pg.43	Crunchy Pepperoni Chips pg.31	Turkey Meatballs pg.37
Tuesday	Almond and Pecan Granola pg.22	Turnip with Chicken Legs pg.39	Zucchini Cheesy Fries pg.32	Old Bay Tuna Patties pg.46
Wednesday	Cheesy Sausage Meatball pg.26	Crunchy Fish Sticks pg.48	Cauliflower Bacon Skewers pg.32	Parmesan Flavored Pork Chops pg.43
Thursday	Avocado and Sausage pg.26	Peppers Stuffed with Sausage pg.44	Crunchy Spinach Chips pg.28	Chicken Burgers with Cheese pg.38
Friday	Chocolate Chip Muffins pg.24	Cauliflower Bacon Skewers pg.32	Pork Belly Vinegar Chips pg.31	Cheese and Herb Flavored Lamb Chops pg.45
Saturday	Pepper and Ham Omelette pg.21	Salmon Kebabs pg.47	Cheesy Pickle Spear pg.31	Chinese Crispy BBQ Duck pg.38
Sunday	Lemon Cake pg.22	Chicken Breast in White Wine pg.37	Avocado French Fries pg.31	Old Bay Tuna Patties pg.46

Conclusion

Congratulations on starting your journey with the ketogenic diet. I'm hoping after making a few recipes, you've realized how satisfying the food is, seen some results, and you've decided to keep going until you reach your fitness goals or to make it a permanent lifestyle change. Whatever you choose to do, here are some tips to keep you on track:

Swap it Out: Most people's kitchen cupboards are filled with high carb, processed and sugary foods, all of which will kick you right out of ketosis and keep you trapped in a cycle of unhealthy eating. When you don't have these options available, you won't eat them. So you can start your keto journey by getting rid of all foods that aren't keto friendly and replacing them with foods that are.

Accountability Partner: Whether you join a Facebook group or you ask a friend to be your accountability partner, make sure you get one. An accountability partner will keep you motivated on the days when you feel like giving up and remind you why you need to keep pushing.

Meal Plan: Meal planning takes some forethought and time but it's a great way to ensure you're getting the right nutrients and controlling your portion sizes. It also relieves you of having to think about what you're going to eat all the time which can cause decision fatigue and will eventually lead to you ditching your diet.

Meal Prep: One of the reasons people revert back to old habits is because they run out of food. When you're hungry and there's nothing in the fridge, the temptation to order a takeaway becomes overwhelming. All it takes is one slip up and you're on a downward spiral of decline. You can avoid this by meal prepping. Meal prepping involves making a lot of food and freezing it in small containers so that you've always got something on hand.

And finally, if you've found this recipe book helpful, I would be really grateful if you could take a few minutes of your time to write a review on Amazon. Reviews are super important because they help others determine whether they want to buy the book. Thank you so much in advance!

Appendix 1 Measurement Conversion Chart

VOLUME EQUIVALENTS (LIQUID)

US STANDARD	US STANDARD OUNCES	METRIC (APPROXIMATE)
1 teaspoon	1/8 fl. oz	5 ml
1 tablespoon	½ fl. oz	15 ml
2 tablespoons	1 fl.oz.	30 ml
1/4 cup	2 fl.oz.	60 ml
1/2 cup	4 fl.oz.	120 ml
1 cup	8 fl.oz	240 ml
1 1/2 cup	12 fl.oz	355 ml
2 cups or 1 pint	16 fl.oz	475 ml
4 cups or 1 quart	32 fl.oz.	1 L
1 gallon	128 fl.oz	4 L

WEIGHT EQUIVALENTS

US STANDARD	METRIC (APPROXIMATE)
1 ounce	28 g
2 ounces	57 g
5 ounces	142 g
10 ounces	284 g
15 ounces	425 g
16 ounces (1 pound)	455 g
1.5 pounds	680 g
2 pounds	907 g

TEMPERATURES EQUIVALENTS

FARENHEIT (F)	CELSIUS(C) (APPROXIMATE)
225° F	107° C
250° F	120° C
275° F	135° C
300° F	150° C
325° F	160° C
350° F	180° C
375° F	190° C
400° F	205° C
425° F	220° C
450° F	235° C
475° F	245° C
500° F	260° C

Limitation of Liability / Disclaimer of Warranty: The publisher and the author of this work are not medical professionals and do not provide medical counseling, treatments, or diagnoses. The contents of this work are provided for informational purposes only and should not be considered a substitute for professional medical advice. The publisher and the author make no warranties or representations regarding the accuracy or completeness of the information presented herein. The information in this work has not been evaluated by the U.S. Food and Drug Administration, and it is not intended to diagnose, treat, cure, or prevent any disease. It is recommended that individuals seek full medical clearance from a licensed physician before initiating any diet or health-related practices. The advice and strategies presented in this work may not be suitable for every individual, and the publisher and the author disclaim any responsibility for any adverse effects or consequences resulting from the use, application, or interpretation of the information provided.

Nutritional Information: The nutritional information provided in this work is based on specific brands, measurements, and ingredients used in the recipes. It is intended for informational purposes only and should not be considered a guarantee of the actual nutritional value of the reader's prepared recipe. The publisher and the author are not responsible for any damages or losses resulting from reliance on the provided nutritional information.